# THE HEALING FATS OF LIFE

BULLETPROOF YOUR HEART, REVERSE MEMORY LOSS AND SUPERCHARGE YOUR IMMUNITY

ALEX BRADFORD

http://www.dailysuperfoodlove.com



Published by Duo Publications

This information is provided as information only and may not be construed as medical advice or instruction. No action should be taken based solely on the contents of this publication. Readers should consult appropriate health professionals on any matter relating to their health and well-being.

The publisher shall not be responsible for errors or omissions.

ISBN: 978-0-6923866-4-4

**Legal Disclaimer**

# CONTENTS

# INTRODUCTION

# THE REAL TRUTH ABOUT THE HEALING POWER OF FATS

Before you begin reading this book, I would like you to do one simple thing.

All I ask is that you suspend disbelief and forget everything you think you know about dietary fats. Everything you have been told by the media, I would like you to forget it.

I know that's asking a lot. However, you now hold in your hands a powerful book that will shatter the lies that have been promoted by the media, powerful commercial players, big Pharma, and governments.

**Fat is not the enemy.**

The plain hard truth is there are thousands of peer-reviewed studies that prove without a doubt that the fat theory was fabricated by various government organizations and commercial industries.

I urge to forget what you think you know about fats. Set your prejudices aside. Don't listen to the mainstream media or well-meaning, old school nutritionists.

I congratulate you for taking the first step to discover for yourself how fat got a bad rap and became entangled in a massive lie.

You see, everyone had it wrong for some time now; there are indeed certain fats that are good for you!

Saturated fats are essential to your health and wellbeing and you can't make them from scratch.

It's only in the last 100 years since humans have figured out how to make oils out of plants like canola (rapeseed), cottonseed, safflower, sunflower, and others. All of a sudden in recent history, nutritionists claim that these man-made oils are more beneficial to your health than natural fats.

What's even worse is that these oils are recommended to reduce heart disease, control cholesterol, and help weight loss. However, these processed oils are high in trans-fats and omega-6 fatty acids, which are linked to inflammation in the body. *Inflammation is the starting point of all chronic diseases from heart disease to cancer.*

Further into this book, I'll share with you clear evidence on how these oils actually create heart disease and increase your risk of life-threatening chronic diseases.

I created this book to help you understand how to use the healing fats of life to supercharge your memory, protect your health, and increase your vitality.

Thank you for taking the time to read it with an open mind.

When I talk about healing fats in this book, I'll discuss several different kinds of fats and how they work to bulletproof your body.

Triglycerides, cholesterol, and other essential fatty acids – the scientific terms for fats your body cannot produce on its own – create hormones, store energy, and protect your vital organs.

Fats also act as messengers, repairmen, and helpers. They create chemical chain reactions that spark growth, immune function, reproduction, and help your cells accumulate vital nutrients such as fat-soluble vitamins A, D, E, & K.

Don't be brainwashed into thinking that eating dietary fat will make you obese or create heart disease. If you or a loved one are suffering from a chronic disease or want to improve your wellbeing in order to add years to your life, this may be the most important book you read.

In the following pages, I'm going to share everything you need to know about how to get the right kinds of fats in your diet and how you can use healing fats to...

**Supercharge your memory** – Find out how you can amplify your brain function, create new neurons, and dramatically lower your risk of developing dementia, Alzheimer's, Parkinson's, and Huntington's disease.

**Add years to your life** – Saturated fat is critical for cellular renewal and optimizes body functions. Without fat, you would cease to function. You'll find out how these healing fats can eradicate free radicals, stop DNA damage, and defend your body against chemical and environmental pollutants.

**Protect your immune system** – These healing fats contain special acids that are essential to your immunity. The number of white blood cells you have directly correlate to the amount of saturated fatty acids in your body.

**Balance hormones** – Eating saturated fat tends to increase free testosterone levels. Why should you care about "free testosterone"? It's huge...it helps with muscle growth, tissue repair, immune system strength, managing weight, and sexual function.

**Bulletproof your heart** – Healing fats can help lower your cholesterol profile and increase good HDL levels. Research shows that saturated fat can slightly raise LDL levels but it also increases the size of the LDL particles. These larger particles are not atherogenic – they do not promote arterial plaque – like smaller particles. It is the smaller ones that you need to worry about, that lead to cardiovascular problems down the road.

Before you dive into the first chapter of the Healing Fats of Life...there is another often-overlooked connection to illness and disease that I want to discuss with you, it is chronic stress.

## How Constant Stress Makes You Sick, Fat, and Miserable

Could you possibly be part of the most "stressed-out" generation of all time?

Stress is so commonplace in our culture that a random search generates hundreds of thousands of results. The American Psychological Association created a study called Stress in America. The study discovered that the average stress level reported by adults in 2012 was 4.9 and the average American believes that 3.6 is a healthy level of stress.

In fact, over 72% of respondents said that their stress level remained the same or increased in the previous five years. Only 20% said their stress level decreased in the previous year.

The stress hormone cortisol – that's critical for survival – is the culprit behind you being so stressed out. Cortisol surges naturally through your body when you're stressed out.

Short-term surges are fine for coping in difficult situations. However, prolonged elevated levels of cortisol that you experience when under constant stress, destroys your body, and suppresses your immune system.

Cortisol is both friend and foe. Prolonged elevated levels of cortisol create inflammation. Since inflammation plays a key role in the onset and progression of nearly all diseases, it is important to understand how elevated stress levels affect your health.

**Long-term stress causes:**

- Anxiety
- Nervousness
- Inflammation
- Weight gain
- Digestion problems
- High blood pressure
- Immune system malfunction
- Heart disease
- Cold and flu
- Allergies
- Slower healing
- Sleep disruption and dysfunction
- Depression
- Chronic Pain

In addition, chronic (ongoing) stress created an environment that caused the body to lose its ability to control and regulate inflammation.

Since inflammation is partly regulated by the hormone cortisol, when cortisol is diverted because the body is under prolonged stress, inflammation can run wild.

Dr. Sheldon Cohen of Carnegie Mellon's Laboratory for the Study of Stress has studied the relationship between stress and disease for 35 years. He said, "When under stress, cells of the immune system are unable to respond to hormonal control and produce levels of inflammation that promote disease."

In three separate studies done by Dr. Cohen's team in 1983, 2006, and 2009 with over 6,300 survey respondents, it was discovered that stress reduced the body's ability to regulate inflammation, which in turn increases short-term memory loss and your chance of developing an illness.

Over the past two decades, scientists have found inflammation to be a direct link to cardiovascular disease, asthma, autoimmune disorders, neurological conditions, infections, and so much more.

Cortisol not only suppresses your immune response, it affects your memory in more ways than you may be aware. It creates increased forgetfulness and interferes with the processes used to store everyday memories.

Which is why you may have experienced short-term memory loss more frequently than you realize. The number one cause behind short-term memory loss and rapidly declining brain function are stress hormones.

As you read the Healing Fats of Life, I want you to use this life-saving information and combine it with small changes in your emotional and mental outlook.

I share with you easy life hacks in the bonuses that can help relieve stress, improve mental performance, and teach you stress resilience.

When you combine the physical, mental, and emotional aspects of health together, you create the ultimate healing solution from the inside out.

The power to prevent threats to your health – and even reverse heart disease, cancer, dementia, and more…all lies within you. *Ready?* Let's get started.

# CHAPTER 1
# HOW FAT GOT A BAD RAP

Around the world, there is a secret hidden in plain sight.

It is as common as the nose on your face. Yet you and I have been trained by society and nutritionists to ignore this health hazard completely.

It's the root cause behind nearly all chronic diseases. It's the problem that keeps mankind fat, sick, and undernourished.

Even if you don't have a weight problem, you can be fooled into thinking that you are not affected by it. *Make no mistake...you are.*

You are sold the lie that fat is bad for you. How did this happen and why is the belief that fat is bad for you so hard to dispel?

Let's take a look at the history of the myth.

Human beings haven't changed much genetically since the beginning of time. Environment, lifestyle, and access to food are what have transformed our society into a sick and overweight population.

Every single day, you are bombarded with the message that "fat is bad, eat more whole grains, eat low fat." Until recently, the Paleo diet, the Ketogenic diet, and even the original Atkins diet were frowned upon as too fatty.

The medical community at large insists that eating more fat will make you sick but that's not the case at all!

## The Dawning of a New Food Era

One of the biggest changes to the way the Western world eats happened in the 1970's. That was when the United States Department of Agriculture (USDA) changed the face of our diet and how the majority of the population would eat from then on. What average people ate and fed their children changed forever.

A man named Earl "Rusty" Butz (yes, that's his real name) was the secretary of the USDA under President Richard Nixon. Butz, an often rude and boisterous man, ruled the farm scene of the United States at that time.

He envisioned an uber-efficient, consolidated food system for America. He had only two requirements: it had to be profitable and cheap.

Butz set about making his dream a reality, installing a program that resembled an iceberg. Seemingly harmless on first sight but carrying devastating consequences on closer inspection.

That iceberg ripped the bottom from beneath the ship of New Deal agricultural policies established by President Roosevelt in the 1930's. The New Deal was initially conceived as a way to help farmers after the Great Depression. President Roosevelt intended the policies to provide farmers with better credit and systems of growing that would ultimately stabilize food prices.

It helped the farmers, it kept our food source local (and purer), and there was competition in the market to ensure prices didn't soar.

All of that changed a few decades later. In 1971, mass-produced "convenience" foods exploded. The entire nation started buying pre-packaged snacks and the fast food industry took a firm foothold within the growing middle class.

The only thing the food industry needed to blaze its trail was a cheap way to produce food. Sugar – lots and lots of cheap sugar – gave them the edge they required. This "fake" food ushered in the era of King Corn and Queen Soy.

Butz envisioned the flood of overgrown Midwestern corn and soy as a way to "feed the world."

At the time, those in charge of agribusiness policies still used restraint. One of the key features of the New Deal was a way to help farmers manage supply and demand. It was important not to promote one crop over another.

Before Butz assumed control of the USDA, farmers left some land fallow and the government paid them to not plant. The following season, the prices for that crop would rise. If the prices rose too high, the payments would stop and planting would begin again. One of the most important goals of the New Deal was to take it easy on the land itself, since the devastating effects of the Depression and the "Dust Bowl" was still fresh in the country's collective memory.

As the new head of the USDA, Butz felt the old way of managing crops was socialism because it stopped the free market. To sell his new method, he had to convince the farmers of the Midwest who grew corn and soy that it would work. He told farmers that if they produced an excess of a specific crop, they'd "sell it overseas!"

In 1973, the last of the New Deal protections in place for American farmers was ripped to shreds by the Farm Bill proposed – and passed – by "Rusty" Butz.

As a result, farmers started churning out more and more corn. Exactly what they'd signed up for wouldn't be apparent for many years.

In the mid 1970's, the food conglomerate Archer Daniel's Midland (ADM) began testing a method originally developed in Japan for producing a concentrated sweetener made from the waste product of corn instead of using harvested sugar.

However, even with corn being overproduced and being sold at bargain basement prices, ADM couldn't make high fructose corn syrup (HFCS) cheaply enough to compete with sugar.

In a diabolical move, ADM convinced the United States Congress to impose a quota on sugar produced in other countries. Imported sugar had kept the price stable but once that was stopped, HFCS became the cheaper option overnight.

Soft drink makers scrambled to switch to ADM's syrup and the production of cheaply made food increased exponentially with the availability of HFCS. According to nutritionist Marion Nestle, this paved the way for obesity.

Food manufacturers quickly embraced the use of high-fructose corn syrup. It was plentiful and cheap. They started adding the industrial sweetener to bread, snack cakes, cookies, breakfast cereal, and more. By the mid 1980's, HFCS replaced sugar in sodas and juices.

The average American consumer's calorie consumption jumped from 3,200 per day in 1970 to 3,900 per day in the early 1980's.

That is nearly twice as much as the human body requires on a daily basis. Far too many of those calories came from sweeteners...and we started getting fat.

## The Great Debate: Fat vs Sugar

In the mid-1970's, while "Rusty" Butz was putting his plan of corn and soy world domination into effect, another fierce debate raged on behind the closed doors of the scientific community.

There are two repercussions from these events that are killing us.

The first health epidemic is obesity.

The population in the Western hemisphere – particularly in the United States – has steadily gotten fatter. This is not about body image, this is about *health*.

Not just "a bit plump." Since the 1960's, the number of people who are considered obese – having a body fat percentage higher than 30 – has *doubled*, increasing from 13.4 to 35.7% in U.S. adults age 20 and older. Another 30% are considered "overweight" – having a body fat percentage higher than 24 but lower than 30.

Among children (age 6-11), obesity hovers around 18% – double what it was three decades ago. Among adolescents (age 12-19), it sits firmly at 21% – triple what it was three decades ago.

That means that more than **two-thirds of our adult population** is considered overweight or obese and **one-third of our child and adolescent population** is overweight or obese.

*Health Risks of Obesity:*

- Type 2 diabetes
- Heart disease
- High blood pressure (hypertension)
- Non-alcoholic fatty liver disease (NAFLD)
- Osteoarthritis
- Some forms of cancer: breast, colon, endometrial, and kidney
- Stroke or heart attack

**What really caused us to get sick and obese - sugar or fat?**

If a calorie was just a calorie, then anything you ate would be processed by your body in the same way...whether its salad, fish, cookies, cakes, protein, sugar, or fat. If all calories were created equal, each one would provide nutrition and adequate fuel.

That isn't how it works because all calories are *not* the same.

The changes in our food supply have become so dangerous that, even if you aren't overweight, it changes your body's biochemical composition.

The average American eats over 90 pounds of sugar per year. The majority of it as an additive to processed foods in the form of high fructose corn syrup – and it is making us incredibly sick.

Your body metabolizes fructose and converts it directly into fat. That is what makes us fatter. When your body is overloaded with sugar, the hormone leptin is suppressed. Leptin is the compound your body uses to tell you that you're full, that you've had enough food, and you should stop eating. Without leptin, your body *never gets the signal* that you are full. You are never truly satiated and you eat too much.

The second health epidemic is heart disease.

What is behind the dramatic rise in heart disease? From the 1930's to the 1950's, infectious diseases were finally being controlled. Antibiotics were effective and with the introduction of penicillin, disease such as TB and the flu dropped.

By the 1950's, one out of every three men in the United States were developing heart disease before the age of sixty. Something needed to be done but the causes of cardiovascular disease were not as widely understood as they are now.

Most scientists believed a preventive approach was better than trying to find a cure.

Enter Dr. Ancel Keys. He developed the army food ration called the K-ration. Dr. Keys believed that fat was the enemy, that fat was the root cause of heart disease, and he presented his findings in the landmark "seven countries" study in 1970.

Back in the 1940s and 1950s, Professor John Yudkin and his colleagues discovered a link between consumption of refined sugar and heart disease. In 1972, Professor Yudkin publicly declared his findings that it was <u>sugar – and not fat – that caused heart disease</u>.

Due to the fact that sucrose (sugar) had only entered the mainstream diet eighty years before, he experienced a backlash of his findings from Ancel Keys. Their feud reached David and Goliath proportions. In the end, Yudkin's work was ultimately discredited and Keys' research on the "danger of fat" prevailed.

<u>Sugar won the battle.</u> As a result, the country continued to consume sugar without any real understanding of the damage it was doing to our bodies.

Even today, sugar is not painted as the villain it truly is.

Sugar consumption lowers your body's resistance to bacteria, viruses, and yeasts that can lead to inflammation in both your heart and arteries. Excess sugar leads to deficiencies in the entire B-vitamin complex, which you need to maintain healthy arteries.

Ongoing research at the U.S. Department of Agriculture indicates that fructose may be even more dangerous than sugar. Fructose, mainly in the form of high-fructose corn syrup (HFCS), has become the sweetener of choice for soft drinks, condiments, and many so-called health foods.

Butz conquered agribusiness with his ideas about corn and soy. Keys won the great debate of fat vs. sugar.

Over 40 years later, we're all paying the price for their "successes" with our health.

A marketing opportunity presented itself to the food industry to create "low-fat" foods that were supposedly heart-healthy and better for you. However, the problem with low-fat foods is that you can't take out the flavor provided by fat and expect the food to taste good. When you remove fat, you create cardboard food. Is there anyone out there that really *likes* the way skim milk tastes?

When the food manufacturers took out the fat, they replaced it with sugar.

The theory behind reduced fat foods is that you can eat more and not get fat. The manufacturers didn't mention that the hidden sugars they added to improve flavor had their own issues. Their products weren't calorie-free!

The average consumer didn't realize that the food they were buying was lab-created, fats were chemically removed, and dangerous sugars were added. The food industry was given "no questions asked" autonomy on our food supply.

Is it any wonder that obesity was a gradually spreading epidemic for forty years?

It turns out that Professor Yudkin was right all along. A new study by Cambridge University, recently published in the *Annals of Internal Medicine*, clearly states that saturated fat does not cause cardiovascular disease.

**The real cause of cardiovascular disease, obesity, diabetes, and even dementia is a high-sugar, high-carb diet.**

The anti-fat campaign gave birth to partially hydrogenated counterparts such as margarine, safflower oil, corn oil, canola oil, and soybean oil that have been promoted – even *pushed* on the population – as the way to go for decades. The campaign has now been proven false!

Dr. Rajiv Chowdhury, lead researcher and author of the study at Cambridge University said, "It's not the saturated fat that we should worry about. It's the high carbohydrate or sugary diet that should be the focus of dietary guidelines."

Dr. Chowdhury and his colleagues drew their conclusions on fat vs sugar from more than 72 published studies of more than 600,000 people from 18 countries around the globe.

In October of 2013, cardiologist Aseem Malhotra turned the nutrition world upside down with his stunning revelation that unprocessed saturated fat is good for you.

Yes, you read that right. **Fat is good for you.**

In the *British Medical Journal*, Dr. Malhotra wrote, "It is time to bust the myth of the role of saturated fat in heart disease and wind back the harms of dietary advice that has contributed to obesity. The food industry has profited from the low-fat mantra for decades because foods that are marketed as low fat are often loaded with sugar. We are now learning that added sugar in food is driving the obesity epidemic and the rise in diabetes and cardiovascular disease."

For nearly four decades, saturated fat had to be cut out of the diet, supposedly to reduce heart disease, while the real culprit was running rampant all along.

Increasing fat in our diets not only stimulates weight loss, it combats epilepsy, reverses type 2 diabetes, prevents Alzheimer's, can reverse ADHD, and most importantly prevents heart disease – the **number one killer** in the Western world.

---

## WHAT IS SATURATED FAT?

"Saturated" fat means that all available carbon atoms are occupied (and fully "saturated") by a hydrogen atom. You can see this in the picture on the right. Unlike unsaturated fats, saturated fats are **highly stable**, and not likely to turn into free radicals or go rancid when exposed to heat, oxygen, or light.

You should be cooking with saturated fats.

---

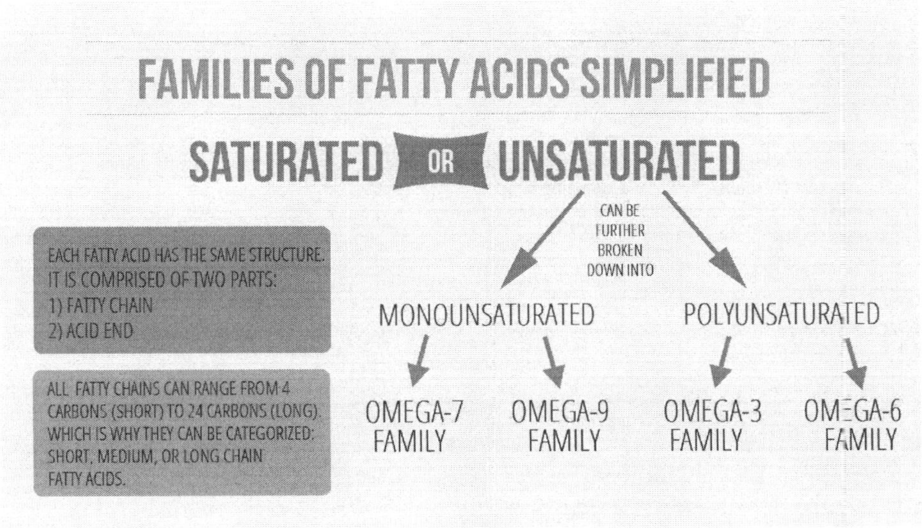


### Why the Types of Dietary Fats You Eat Matter

Are you always on a diet or do you know someone who is? Do they obsessively count fat grams? It's time to put a stop to it.

Here's the truth. The percentage of calories that come from the fat you eat doesn't matter. What matters is the *type* of dietary fat you eat.

Also, let's look at the labels – "low fat," "reduced fat," "good fats," "bad fats," or "fat-free." For most of your life, I am sure it has been drilled into your subconscious, "Low-fat is best."

No doubt, you have heard this well-meaning but misguided advice, "A reduced-fat diet will protect your heart and lower your cholesterol." Well nothing could be further from the truth. Low fat diets are often high in sugar, refined carbohydrates, and offer no nutritional value. We will dig into and uncover the truth about fats in the following chapters.

**100 Calories of Margarine vs. 100 Calories of Grass-Fed Butter**

Margarine contains vegetable oil, emulsifiers, colorants, and various unknown artificial ingredients. One tablespoon or 100 calories of margarine contains 3 grams of trans fat and 2 grams of saturated fat.

Since vegetable oil is liquid at room temperature, margarine must be "hydrogenated" to give it a shelf life and make it stable. This turns some of vegetable oils into trans fats. Margarine is full polyunsaturated omega-6 fatty acids. Several studies link polyunsaturated vegetable oils with inflammation, cancer, heart disease, and even violent behavior. Trans fat raises LDL (bad) cholesterol and also lowers HDL (good) cholesterol that prevents artery plaque.

Butter is made from the cream of cow's milk. One tablespoon or 100 calories of butter contains 7 grams of saturated fat.

The fatty portion known as heavy cream, double cream, or heavy whipping cream is agitated until it turns into the final product...butter.

Always choose organic grass-fed butter or cream. Cows naturally eat grass, but on many industrial farms, they are fed grain-based feeds. This affects the nutritional content.

Grass fed butter is packed with vitamin K2, CLA an anti-cancer nutrient, butyrate fights inflammation, and omega-3 heart protective fatty acid.

---

Here's a fun little experiment. Take one empty Mason jar and fill the jar halfway with the heavy cream, screw on the lid, and shake it (shake from lid to bottom, not side to side) or give to a kid to shake for about five minutes.

In two minutes, you will have whipped cream, in another 3 minutes you'll have butter. Once you open the jar, you will see a yellow clump of butter and some thin liquid.

Discard the buttermilk and place the butter (large and small chunks) into a bowl. Add a cup of cold water and knead the butter together into a ball. This removes the buttermilk and you will now have fresh butter. Put it in a clean bowl and let it sit in the fridge, you now have delicious vitamin packed butter!

---

A Meta study in March 2009 by the American Society for Nutrition of 21 separate studies and 37,747 subjects was compiled that evaluated the association of saturated fat with cardiovascular disease, stroke, and coronary heart disease.

The results of the findings showed that there was NO significant evidence for concluding that dietary saturated fat is associated with increased risk of cardiovascular disease, stroke, and coronary heart disease.

Saturated fat doesn't create heart disease or block your arteries it doesn't even contribute to it.

Margarine on the other hand was linked to heart disease in 4 different studies examined in the Meta study. Trans fats and poly-unsaturated vegetable oils were also associated with cardiovascular disease and death in 3 different studies examined in the Meta study.

**What Are Trans Fats?**

Trans fats are fats that have been chemically changed to have a longer shelf life. When you heat unsaturated fat at high temperature with hydrogen gas, it is converted to a "trans fat."

The entire process combines high pressure, high heat, hydrogen gas, and metal catalyst.

In the case of trans fat, the oil ends up with a bit of the hydrogen in the end product. That's why the term on the label is "partially hydrogenated" – for that little bit that remains. This process also mutates the bonds – carbon atoms – that form the fat.

In one study after another, trans fats have been linked to learning disorders, behavior disorders, immune system decline, toxicity in the liver, advanced aging, chronic disease, weight gain, and chromosomal mutation.

Trans fats inhibit the production of prostaglandin – a hormone that regulates the contraction of muscle, blood vessels, blood pressure, and inflammation. Not having adequate levels of prostaglandin in your blood can lead to blood clots and the increased risk of myocardial infarction or a heart attack – where the blood flow to your heart is suddenly interrupted and cannot deliver necessary oxygen to the heart muscle.

While the United States Food and Drug Administration (FDA) have "restricted" the use of trans fats, they have not cracked down on all the *loopholes* that food manufacturers use to get around the regulations. If any product you're buying contains "partially hydrogenated" anything – then you're getting trans fats. Possibly, in trace amounts...but you're getting them.

*Bottom line: trash the margarine and trans-fats - reach for healthy saturated fats instead.*

# CHAPTER 2
# SURPRISE! YOUR BODY CRAVES FAT

Your body functions better with fat. Does that shock you?

Science is only *now* beginning to understand the role that fat plays in our bodies. Since fat was cast as the villain in the United States as far back as the late 1950's, it's no wonder that most Americans equate "low-fat" with "healthy."

The fat-phobia has to stop. If the low-fat diet actually showed results in reducing the obesity epidemic, it might hold water. It doesn't help at all.

In fact, countless studies have proven that your body *craves* fat.

In order to understand this counterintuitive concept (and what feels plain *wrong* to most of us), you have to grasp the biology behind your body's need for fat and what it is that fat does for you.

The body can't make triglycerides, cholesterol, and other essential fatty acids – responsible for creating critical chemical reactions, producing hormones, regulating your metabolism, maintaining immune function, storing energy, as well as insulating and protecting your vital organs – so the presence of fat is key to your biology.

Fat is necessary for your *survival.*

Fat is a source of energy for your body and acts as a potent detoxifier. When a chemical or toxin enters your system, your body attempts to neutralize the threat by storing it in adipose (fat) tissue.

Chemically speaking, all fats are made up of varying number of hydrogen, oxygen, and carbon atoms arranged in different orders. Each carbon atom is bonded to two other carbon atoms. The more carbon atoms present in a given fatty acid, the longer the chain will be.

Fatty acids with longer chains typically have higher melting points and yield more energy when metabolized.

**Fats can be categorized into four main types:**

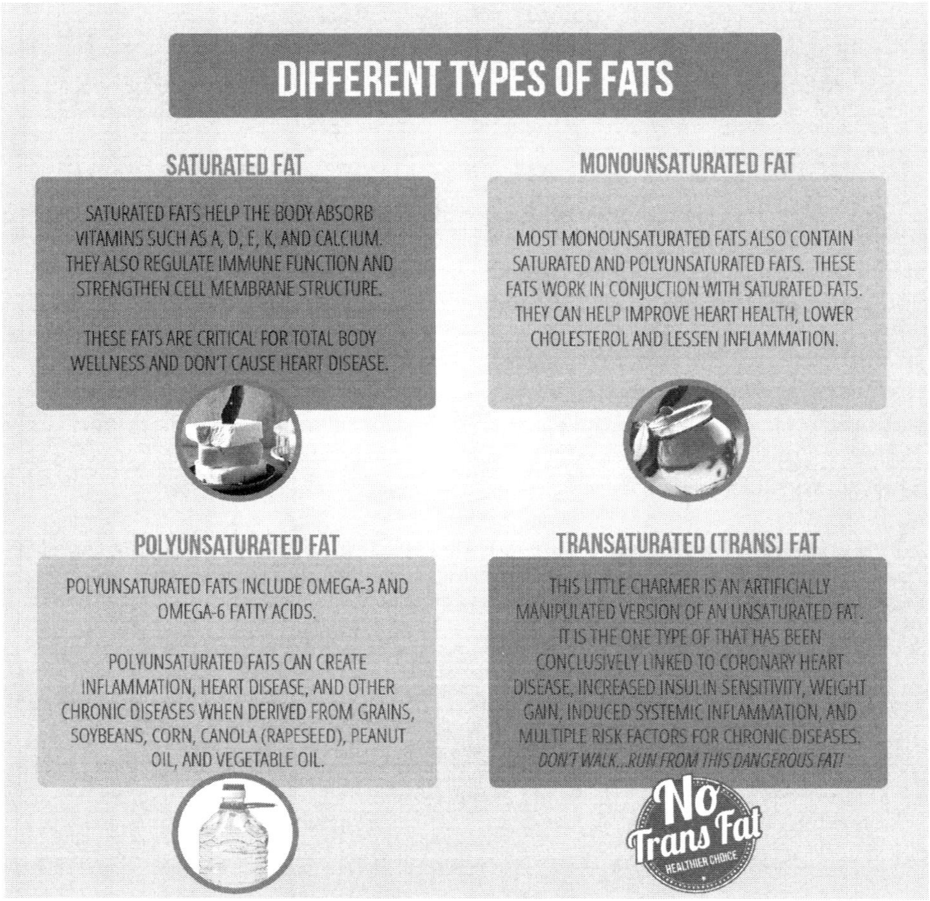


**Saturated Fat:** Each carbon atom is bonded to two hydrogen atoms, meaning that each carbon molecule is "saturated" with hydrogen. These fats are often solid at room temperature. They are found in red meat, tallow, lard, whole milk products, butter, ghee, suet, tallow, palm oil, coconut oil, and cacao.

Saturated fats help the body absorb vitamins such as A, D, E, K, and calcium. They also regulate immune function and strengthen cell membrane structure. These fats are critical for total body wellness and don't cause heart disease.

We're going to dig deeper into why you shouldn't let the term "saturated fat" scare you.

**Monounsaturated Fat:** Each carbon atom is bonded to only one hydrogen atom and double bonded to another carbon. They are found in tree nuts, sesame, flax, peanut, sunflower, olives, and avocados. <u>Most monounsaturated fats also contain saturated and polyunsaturated fats</u>.

Olive oil is a monounsaturated fat and it is praised by the medical and nutrition communities.

You need to use these types of fats in moderation and avoid heating them to high temperatures. Olive oil begins to break down once it is heated over 200 degrees Fahrenheit and begins to unleash free radicals that lead to disease.

**Polyunsaturated Fat:** Contains more than one of the double bonds within the carbon chain. These fats include omega-3 and omega-6 fatty acids. They can be found in grains, soybeans, corn, canola (rapeseed), peanut oil, vegetable oil, flax seed oil, tung oil, poppy seed oil, and walnut oil.

Polyunsaturated fats remain liquid even at cooler temperatures, go rancid easily, and break down into free radicals when heated. Most people and almost all fast food restaurants reach for these oils when frying food so the chances are high that you've consumed them whether you know it or not. Frying requires extremely high heat and these oils break down quickly, unleashing free radicals into your body.

**Transaturated (Trans) Fat:** This little charmer is an artificially manipulated version of an unsaturated fat. It is the one type of fat that has been conclusively linked to coronary heart disease. You'll find it in baking shortenings, shortenings used to manufacture industrial baked goods, for deep-frying in restaurants, and margarines.

In one study published in the *Division of Cardiovascular Medicine*, Brigham and Women's Hospital - Harvard Medical School found that consuming trans-fat or trans-fatty acids adversely affects cardiovascular health.

Trans-fatty acids also worsened insulin sensitivity, stimulated weight gain, increased pro-inflammatory markers, induced systemic inflammation, and is linked to multiple risk factors for chronic diseases.

Don't walk...*run* from this dangerous artificial fat!

*Note:* Although most trans-fats are artificial, there are naturally-occurring trans fats that are actually healthy - like the CLA (conjugated linoleic acid) found in grass-fed beef, dairy, and butter. CLA is a trans-rumeric fatty acid, "rumeric" means it comes from grass eating "ruminant" animals.

## Leveling the Playing Field

Not all fats are created equal – just like calories. Don't let the fat haters with their mind-numbing advice of "eliminate the fat in your diet," stop you from experiencing how the **right types of fat** can transform your health.

Saturated fat found in foods such as fatty meats, coconut oil, butter, organic lard, and ghee *will not make you fat*.

In fact, these types of fats will heal your body and help you perform at an optimal level.

## Why Your Body Craves the "Amazing Functions" of Fat:

Prevent Cardiovascular Disease: In 1992, Dr. William Castelli, a former director of the Framingham Heart Study, stated...

> *"In Framingham, Massachusetts, the more saturated fat one ate, the more cholesterol one ate, the more calories one ate, the lower the person's serum cholesterol. The opposite of what Keys et al would predict. We found that the people who ate the most cholesterol, ate the most saturated fat, ate the most calories, weighed the least and were the most physically active."*

*Saturated fat reduced levels of a substance found in LDL (bad) cholesterol called lipoprotein (a) (Lp(a)) that correlates strongly with the risk for heart disease. As of now, there are no medications available on the market to lower this substance and the dietary means of lowering Lp(a) is by eating saturated fat. In addition, eating saturated fat also raises your level of high-density lipoproteins (HDL) or "good" cholesterol.*

Protect Your Brain: *Your brain is 60% fat. As a matter of fact, your brain is mainly composed of fat, triglycerides, and more cholesterol than any other organ in your body.* The brain cell membranes need fat to carry messages more quickly to various nerve fibers. Fat also insulates the protective sheath around these fibers.

The brain is composed of two major fats – saturated and a fat called arachidonic acid. Saturated fats like butter, tallow, lard, coconut oil, and meat fats are the kinds of fats your brain wants.

The lesser-known fat of arachidonic acid is a type of omega-6 fat that's found in only butter, egg yolks, organ meats, and meat fats. Arachidonic acid also controls inflammation.

Your brain is 11% arachidonic acid, so when the health establishment is telling you to eat egg-white omelets, you're losing out on the yolks that provide critical fat needed for optimal brain function. The best source of arachidonic acid is butter, liver, and egg yolks. We will go in depth on how you can create a fat-fueled bulletproof brain in chapter five.

Improve Liver Health: Saturated fat lowers the incidence of non-alcohol fatty liver disease (NAFLD). It encourages the liver cells to get rid of fat cells so the liver can function more efficiently. Even a diet that's very high in saturated fat (about 60% of total calories) does not cause fatty liver disease.

Build Stronger Bones**:** When bone mass starts to decline in middle age, the first thing you might reach for are calcium supplements. Before you start to double up on the calcium, did you know that saturated fat is required for calcium to be absorbed effectively into bone? Dr. Mary Enig, PhD, a leading researcher on dietary fat and human health, suggests that nearly 50% of the fats in your diet should be saturated for this reason alone.

Balance Hormones**:** Eating saturated fat increases "free testosterone" levels. Why should you care about "free testosterone?" It's huge and most people have never heard of it. Free testosterone helps with muscle growth, tissue repair, immune system strength, managing weight, and sexual function, you can find out about it in chapter eight.

Retain Omega-3 Fatty Acids**:** Mary Enig, a pioneer in coconut oil research, discovered that when you increase the amount of saturated fat in your diet, you don't need as much fish oil. In fact, when fat levels are up you convert the eicosapentaenoic acids (EPA) into their usable form docosahexaenoic acid (DHA). DHA keeps your brain and vision sharp.

Strengthen Your Immune System**:** In the *Healing Fats of Life*, you'll find out what makes coconut oil so special and absolutely critical to your total health. Coconut oil contains a special acid called lauric acid. This acid is essential to your immunity.

Lauric acid is found in breast milk. Human breast milk is over 54% lauric acid (monolaurin). This "first food" provides the basis for your immune system at the beginning of life. Your white blood cell count directly correlates to the amount of saturated fatty acids in your body. Lower saturated fatty acids in lymphocytes are responsible for the age-related decline in white blood cell function.

Cell Renewal**:** Fat is vital to cell health. Surrounding each cell membrane in your body is a layer of fat. Without that fat, we would cease to function. Fat is also used to build new cells and nerves.

Healthy Hair & Glowing Skin**:** Fat preserves strong hair and skin. Saturated fat helps absorb increased amounts of vitamin A, D, E, and K through the bloodstream. If you have dry flaky skin, it may be a symptom of a deficiency in fatty acids.

**Fat is a great multitasker and the right kinds of fat are vitamin carriers.**

Recent science backs up Dr. Weston Price's findings. These hidden vitamins are found in grass-fed animals (in their fat and organ meat), wild seafood, (free range or pastured) eggs, and oily fish.

Vitamin A**:** This vitamin is essential for mineral and protein metabolism. It is required to prevent birth defects and aids in the healthy development of infants and children. Vitamin A also protects you against infection, aids in the production of stress hormones, and keeps your eyes healthy.

Vitamin D**:** Protects bones, your central nervous system, muscle tone, reproductive health, and insulin production. It also helps you metabolize essential vitamins and minerals, protects against depression, and prevents cancer and heart disease.

Vitamin K2**:** Plays an important role in growth and facial development, healthy teeth and bones, prevents inflammation of the arteries, and increases learning capabilities.

You can amplify these vitamin carriers with whole foods. Whip up a plate of delicious scrambled eggs with two handfuls of fresh spinach cooked in coconut oil. You'll get vitamins E, D, and A from the spinach. Thanks to saturated fat in the coconut oil and eggs, the vitamin A will be converted to retinol. Not to mention, boost your immune system and reverse aging.

# CHAPTER 3

# THE ASTONISHING SCIENCE OF THE HEALING FAT: COCONUT OIL

Imagine you are on a breezy tropical island. The sun warms your face as you stand with your feet firmly planted in soft pink sand. You drink fresh coconut water from a fallen green coconut. You stare out into the expanse of clear turquoise water.

You decide to lie down, close your eyes, and begin to drift off into a peaceful afternoon nap, when suddenly your cell phone rings. It's your boss telling you that you're needed back in the office immediately. Your idyllic vacation is over. It's back to fluorescent lighting and sitting for hours on end in front of a computer screen without moving a muscle.

Instead of drinking delicious coconut water while you enjoy the beach, you're stressed out, sipping a chemical-laden energy drink, and eating genetically modified Franken-food out of a greasy paper bag.

As you try to forget your vacation and focus on work, you start to feel a throbbing pain in your neck, you notice your pants are a bit tighter than they were last month, your skin looks sallow, and you feel like a battery drained of its energy.

*How can you look and feel your best within the confines of your daily routine?*

The answer lies in the saturated healing fat of coconut oil. Let's examine how virgin coconut oil is one of the best healing fats of life. It helps you stay alert, keeps you trim and healthy, protects your brain, bulletproofs your heart, and boosts your immune system.

It may be difficult at times to accept that saturated fat is good for you after almost forty years of the mass media droning on about the benefits of low fat and low cholesterol diets.

Keep reading to discover the proof for yourself

## A Disease-Free Native Population that Thrived on Coconut Oil

In 1989, one of the last civilizations on Earth that had dietary habits closest to our ancestors was extensively studied. The inhabitants of a little island called Kitava; one of the Trobriand Islands in Papua, New Guinea.

The famous Malinowski study found that of the 23,000 people living on the island, there were no indications of heart disease, obesity, high blood pressure, dementia, stroke, or diabetes. The Kitavans remained physically active and vital into their late 80's and 90's. The question researchers wanted to know was fairly simple.

*What were the Kitavans eating that was so different?*

Their primary diet consists of root vegetables, banana, pineapple, watermelon, tropical fruits, coconut, and fish. Less than .2% of their diet comes from dairy, sugar, grains, or alcohol.

What is truly remarkable is their saturated fat consumption. Due to the large quantity of coconut in their daily diets, approximately 30% of their diet is made up of saturated fat from coconuts.

Yet there were no indications of stroke, diabetes, dementia, or congestive heart failure found in the natives of Kitava. The inhabitants are not overweight, don't suffer from acne, or have high blood pressure.

Modern science is finally catching up to what the Kitavans have known for centuries.

Saturated fat doesn't cause chronic disease and it doesn't hurt your heart.

In reality, the food pyramid created by the U.S. government in the 1980's is absolutely ridiculous. It is the 11 servings of rice and pasta per day and absence of fat that set the stage for widespread heart disease. It remains the number one killer in the country and obesity is out of control.

> *"It is time to bust the myth of the role of saturated fat in heart disease and wind back the harms of dietary advice that has contributed to obesity."*

## Time to Bust Three Widespread Myths about Coconut Oil

### MYTH #1

**Since coconut oil is a saturated fat, even though it can help prevent dementia, it can cause heart disease.**

**Myth Buster:** Native populations from the Kitavans to the Veddas (the "Forest People" of Sri Lanka) have virtually no incidences of coronary heart disease.

A study examined 207 adults from age 20-83 years of age. A complete physical examination was taken of each subject, with an emphasis on cardiac health. Electrocardiograms (ECG's) were conducted and no cases of heart disease were found in any of the subjects. Their triglyceride levels and blood cholesterol were normal. HDL (good cholesterol that protects against heart disease) is excellent.

Like the Kitavans, the coconut palm is a primary food source for the Veddas. The majority of their diet comes from coconut and wild game, both of which are high in saturated fat.

The average Vedda consumes an equivalent of **30 quarts of coconut oil** per year.

If coconut oil caused or even *increased the risk* of heart disease, it would be evident in the general population of these two locations. In the United States – where coconut oil consumption is less than one percent – the majority of the population consumes soybean and other polyunsaturated oils, the heart attack death rate is 280 times higher!

### MYTH #2

**MCT Oil (fractionated coconut oil or medium chain triglyceride oil) is better than natural coconut oil.**

**Myth Buster:** Natural coconut oil contains **10 fatty acids**, 63% of which are medium chain or short fatty acids.

When MCT oil is produced, it is divided into different fatty acids. MCT oil consists of only two medium chain fatty acids (MCFAs) – caprylic and capric acid. The most important fatty acid – lauric acid – is removed. Lauric acid is an antiviral that boosts the immune system.

Although MCT oil is beneficial, natural coconut oil offers increased benefits of antimicrobial lauric acid, improved HDL levels, correction of fasting blood glucose levels, reduction in waist circumference, and a decrease in the C-reactive protein (CRP) – a marker for inflammation and heart disease.

# MYTH #3

## It doesn't matter what type of coconut oil you choose. All coconut oil is the same.

**Myth Buster:** Coconut oil processing varies by manufacturer. Refined coconut oil can begin with "copra" or dried coconut and goes through a process known as "RBD," which stands for **r**efined, **b**leached, and **d**eodorized.

| Type of Coconut Oil | Rating Scale 1 to 10 | |
|---|---|---|
| Hydrogenated Coconut Oil | 0 | DO NOT USE |
| Liquid Coconut Oil | 1 | Missing lauric acid |
| Refined, Bleached, and Deodorized | 4 | Chemical residue |
| Refined Physical Coconut Oil | 6 | Good |
| Fresh Pressed Virgin Coconut Oil | 8 | Very Good |
| Wet-Milled, No Heat, Virgin Coconut Oil | 9 | Excellent |
| Wet-Mill Fermented, Heated Virgin Coconut Oil | 10 | The Ultimate Best |

Avoid copra-produced coconut oils. They do not contain the original whole food properties of coconut and may have gone through chemical refining that uses solvent extracts.

Also, avoid hydrogenated coconut oils. Hydrogenated coconut oil is not found in nature and contains trans fats. Refined, bleached, and deodorized coconut oil made from "copra" is processed further to create hydrogenated coconut oil. Always avoid hydrogenated coconut oil. This creates a coconut oil not found in nature, which contains trans fats. Hydrogenated coconut oil also stays unnaturally solid at temperatures higher than 76 degrees F.

**Is coconut oil the superior choice to increase nutrient absorption?**

Many doctors and editors of health journals are frequently shouting that there is insufficient evidence to support the claims about coconut oil. Even bestselling authors, with credentials a mile long, have asked this particular question.

There have been over 17,000 studies done on coconut oil, when you take various terms and components into account.

- Virgin Coconut Oil
- Medium Chain Fatty Acids
- Medium Chain Triglycerides
- Lauric Acid
- Capric Acid
- Caprylic Acid

Even subtracting duplicate studies, that is still more than 10,000 studies!

*Ten thousand studies done on* any topic *should provide enough "sufficient evidence" for anyone, don't you agree?*

Particularly when you consider that the FDA gives approvals to new drugs with only **two positive studies** published. That's right – just two studies are enough to get FDA approval on pharmaceutical drugs!

The basic chemistry of coconut oil was figured out back in the 1920s. Researchers knew then that it was special and radically different from other fats and oils. The unique family of fats found in coconut oil is composed of medium chain fatty acids. In coconut oil, these fatty acids are in the form of medium chain triglycerides (MCTs).

In its purest state, coconut oil has no cholesterol and is free of trans fats. In its non-hydrogenated state, it is packed with medium chain fatty acids.

Your body *loves* coconut oil because it is easily broken down to be used for immediate fuel.

- 91% saturated fatty acids (65% of those saturated fats are in the form of medium chain fatty acids)
- 6% mono-unsaturated fatty acids
- 3% poly-unsaturated fatty acids

These specific medium chain triglycerides (MCTs) make coconut oil unique from all other saturated fats.

The health benefits are proven in one study after another. Doctors and scientists have discovered that this abundant and inexpensive product has incredible versatility...from a skin cream to an Alzheimer's treatment.

Take a look at just five ways coconut oil can restore nutrient balance, increase vitamin absorption, and supercharge cellular activity:

- In the 1930s, researchers at Auburn University studied the effects of B-1 (thiamine) deficiency. Lacking this vitamin leads to a fatal cardiovascular disease called beriberi and can affect the metabolism, brain neurotransmitters, amino acid production, and neuromodulation.

- When rats were given a vitamin B-deficient diet and fed coconut oil, it prevented the disease and made what little of the vitamin that was in the diet more biologically available.
- Researchers at Kerala University in India discovered that coconut oil improves the absorption of not only fat-soluble vitamins but also vitamins A, D, beta-carotene, CoQ10, calcium, magnesium, and some amino acids.
- One study compared the effects of coconut oil versus safflower oil regarding the absorption of carotenoids from tomatoes. The coconut oil performed much better due to the large proportion of medium chain fatty acids it contains.
- Coconut oil is a standard ingredient in most commercial infant formulas due to its ability to promote faster weight gain, growth, and improved nutrient absorption in babies.

## Coconut Oil the Healing Fat of Life

### LIVING PROOF FROM THE COCONUT RESEARCH CENTER OPERATED BY BRUCE FIFE, N.D

Coconut oil is helping thousands of people with various health problems. Here is one fascinating example of the benefits it offers.

*I was once diagnosed with lupus, lichen planus (lost all 20 nails), ADD (attention deficit disorder), depression, COPD (chronic obstructive pulmonary disease), allergies, atherosclerosis (hardening of the arteries) with chest pain, metabolic syndrome, rapidly progressing to full blown diabetes, high CRP (inflammation), high cholesterol, high triglycerides, chronic fatigue, and fibromyalgia," said Peggy M.*

*"I was living on inhalers, antibiotics, prednisone, antidepressants, sleeping pills, allergy meds and more. I began to try alternative things. I am sooooo thankful to say, I have been using organic coconut oil for several years. My thyroid meds continue to be decreased, and I no longer have to take any allergy meds besides shots. I'm afraid to quit them. My breathing problems are totally gone. I have healthy nails, no fibromyalgia, metabolic syndrome, or diabetes.*

**Coconut oil is truly the healing fat of life.**

Coconut oil contains several key nutrients and acids that have the power to keep you free of heart disease, cancer, diabetes, and many of the chronic health conditions we face daily. These nutrients are the key to revitalizing your DNA and renewing your cells.

Today most of us get these nutrients in limited quantities. Even though we consume more than ever before in history, the human population – even in the "developed" world – is sadly undernourished.

Now there's more exciting news…

Coconut oil is finally in the spotlight. Recent studies reveal how coconut oil can heal your body and help you successfully:

- Treat allergies
- Shed fat and help you stay slim
- Reduce pain (including pain from inflammation and osteoarthritis)
- Boost your immunity
- Supercharge your metabolism
- Prevent Alzheimer's disease, senility, and dementia
- Provide stress relief
- Prevent gum disease and tooth decay
- Relieve depression and reverse ADHD
- Fight and prevent certain types of cancer
- Reverse heart disease and lower cholesterol
- Treat cold and flu symptoms
- Clear up acne and reverse wrinkles
- Treat wounds, fungal and yeast infections
- Regulate blood sugar and blood pressure levels
- Activate essential vitamins

When I discuss coconut oil, I'm always referring to **virgin coconut oil** even though I simply say "coconut oil."

## The Essential Building Blocks of Coconut Oil: Medium Chain Triglycerides (MCTs)

Coconut oil is the most natural saturated fat known to mankind. It is 92% saturated and solid at room temperature. Technically, you could call it "coconut fat" instead of "coconut oil."

In comparison, other vegetable oils are only around 15% saturated, lard (from beef fat) is 50% saturated, and butter is 63% saturated.

The special structure of coconut oil is what gives it its unique healing properties. Coconut oil is 60% medium chain triglycerides (MCT) and only 40% long chain triglycerides (LCT).

MCTs are digested differently than other fats. They're transported directly from your intestine to your liver for fuel. The liver rapidly metabolizes these types of fatty acids and burns them for energy.

They are also more likely to be burned for fuel rather than deposited as fat on your waistline. Your body burns MCFAs for energy except, unlike carbohydrates, they don't raise blood sugar or insulin levels.

The fatty acids in coconut oil are 12 carbon atoms or shorter. Corn, soy, and canola oil have almost no short or medium chain fatty acids.

Research from McGill University in Canada suggests that medium chain fatty acids or medium chain triglycerides (MCTs) can boost metabolism, increase satiety, prevent infections, stimulate thyroid function, and provide complete nourishment for our bodies.

Medium chain fatty acids protect against heart disease and lower cholesterol. In addition, the differences in the way MCTs are processed by the body make them ideal to treat a number of medical conditions.

Extensive Clinical Research on MCTs to Treat:

- Cystic fibrosis
- Accelerate recovery after intestinal surgery
- Weight management
- Pancreatic insufficiency
- Metabolic disorders
- Neurological disorders, Alzheimer's, Parkinson's, and dementia
- Treat parasites
- Epilepsy
- Colitis
- Gallbladder disease

*When researchers compared the fatty acid composition of the phospholipids in white blood cells from young and old donors, they found that a loss of saturated fatty acids was responsible for age-related declines in white blood cell functions.*

Saturated fatty acids are also needed for signaling and stabilization processes in the body. When these saturated fatty acids are not available, certain growth factors in your cells and organs will not be properly aligned. The different receptors need to be coupled with lipids in order provide localization of function.

Coconut oil is predominately a medium chain triglyceride oil (63%), which means, "The biological effects of coconut oil are a consequence of the presence of these acids," stated Hans Kaunitz, MD, professor of pathology at Columbia University Medical School and longtime MCT researcher.

## How to Choose the Right Coconut Oil

The quality of the coconut oil you choose is important. When we talk about coconut oil, we always mean **"extra virgin organic coconut oil."**

Brands on the market use various production methods, some of which limit and can even cancel the benefits of using this natural wonder. Make sure you check your labels!

Coconut oil in its purest state has no cholesterol and is free of trans fats. In its non-hydrogenated state, it is packed with medium chain fatty acids. Your body loves coconut oil because it is easily broken down and used for immediate fuel.

If you select "refined" coconut oil – you will be using a product that has gone through several manufacturing processes. It has no scent because it is bleached and deodorized.

Refined coconut oil doesn't use fresh coconut but kernels that have been dried and stored for an undetermined and often unstated length of time.

The difference between buying "unrefined" or "extra virgin" coconut oil is easy to see, smell, and taste. There should be a light coconut flavor and scent, it will be white in color, and have a creamy texture at room temperature.

Unrefined oils are made from fresh coconuts, but you still have to watch the processing methods to determine the right product for you. Refined oils are cheaper and easier to find, but unrefined "virgin" oils are worth the slightly higher cost.

I've discovered that the best coconut oils list the words: raw, organic, and extra virgin on the label. **They are processed from fresh raw coconuts that use a wet milling process.**

Never buy coconut oil extracted from dried coconut, also known as "copra," which could be processed with chemical solvents.

Refined, bleached, and deodorized coconut oil made from "copra" is processed further to create hydrogenated coconut oil. Always avoid hydrogenated coconut oil. This creates a coconut oil not found in nature, which contains trans fats. Hydrogenated coconut oil also stays unnaturally solid at temperatures higher than 76 degrees F.

Choosing the right coconut oil means it is raw, virgin, organic, 100% non-toxic, and has all the health benefits to supercharge your health starting now.

## COCONUT OIL DOSAGE CHART

Coconut oil is safe for people of all ages, but check with your child's pediatrician for exact dosage based on their age and weight.

For newborns, the application of coconut oil through breastfeeding should be sufficient if it is reapplied throughout the day.

This is a general guideline! Coconut oil is non-toxic so it would be almost impossible to overdose on it. However, too much may lead to loose stools – and that is no fun for anyone.

COCONUT OIL HUMAN DOSAGE CHART

- Age 12 – 24: 1 to 1½ tablespoons per day.
- Age 25 – 34: 1½ to 2 tablespoons per day.
- Age 35 – 44: 2 to 2½ tablespoons per day.
- Age 45 – 54: 2½ to 3 tablespoons per day.
- Age 55 – 69: 3 to 3½ tablespoons per day.
- Age 70 years and up: 4 tablespoons per day.

COCONUT OIL PET DOSAGE CHART

- 1 teaspoon per day per 10 pounds of bodyweight or
- 1 tablespoon per 30 pounds of bodyweight

**ALWAYS REMEMBER TO START SLOW AND EASE YOUR WAY UP TO THE RECOMMENDED DOSE.**

## CHAPTER 4

# SUPERCHARGE YOUR IMMUNE SYSTEM WITH THE MOTHER OF ALL ANTIVIRALS

One of the elements that make coconut oil so special is its unique composition of medium chain triglycerides (MCTs) and nearly 50% of its MCTs are lauric acid.

Fatty acids such as lauric acid with 8 to 12 carbon chains in length are naturally more antiviral.

### The "First Food" of Life Found in Coconut Oil

Our bodies convert lauric acid into the substance monolaurin. The only other source of monolaurin in the world is human breast milk.

From birth, the human body is equipped to protect a newborn with the highest level of antiviral protection since their immune system isn't yet fully developed.

Studies on lauric acid derived from virgin coconut oil added to breast milk or formula was found to increase protection around the infant's nose, ears, eyes, and mouth, which are especially vulnerable to infections and pathogens.

Approximately 3.5% of the caloric content in human breast milk is lauric acid. Coconut oil offers double the protection, with 7% of the caloric content represented by lauric acid.

### Treat Your Skin Conditions Naturally

Around the world, severe skin infections are broadly treated with systemic antibiotics that can cause serious side effects and allergic reactions. Drug resistance due to overuse of antibiotics is making it harder and harder to treat conditions that were once under control.

The fact that no new antibiotics are being developed because they aren't "money makers" to the pharmaceutical companies means that our options to fight viruses, bacteria, and fungi are becoming limited in the traditional medical community.

By treating skin infections with natural choices such as coconut oil, you avoid having to flood your body with antibiotics yet again. Coconut oil researchers have confirmed that this incredible product possesses antimicrobial, antiviral, and antiprotozoal properties that are comparable to the effectiveness of standard medicine.

In some cases, coconut oil performs even *better*.

**The lauric acid in coconut oil is converted into monolaurin –the mother of all antivirals. It is naturally antifungal, antibacterial, and an immune system booster.**

In clinical studies, monolaurin killed pathogens including respiratory syncytial virus (RSV), herpes simplex virus type 1 (HSV-1), Haemophilus influenza, salmonella, and Group B streptococcus.

Although these claims are finally being extensively studied, we already have a mountain of evidence proving that coconut oil is extremely effective in killing bacteria and is one of the greatest antivirals known to humankind.

**Viruses and Bacteria Inactivated by Monolaurin**

Viruses

- Human immunodeficiency virus HIV-1 or HIV+
- Measles virus
- Herpes simplex virus-1 (HSV-1)
- Vesicular stomatitis virus (VSV)
- Visna virus
- Cytomegalovirus (CMV)
- Influenza virus
- Pneumonovirus
- Syncytial virus
- Rubeola virus

Bacteria

- Listeria monocytogenes
- Staphylococcus aureus
- Streptococcus agalactiae
- Groups A,B,F & G streptococci
- Gram-positive organisms
- Gram-negative organisms if pretreated with chelator

That's not all, in his study of coconut oil properties, Dr. Joseph Mercola found that coconut oil could destroy viruses coated in lipid (fat) such as herpes, influenza, nearly all pathogenic bacteria, and even HIV.

With antibiotic resistant bacteria multiplying exponentially, we need a substance that can resist infections and help us stay healthy in the age of *Methicillin-resistant Staphylococcus aureus* (MRSA) – a dangerous strain of staph bacteria that has mutated and is now resistant to every antibiotic we have to fight it. MRSA is found on the skin and in the mucus membranes of as much as **one-third of the population**!

Since it was first discovered in 1961, MRSA is frighteningly common. Half of all *Staph aureus* infections in the U.S. are resistant to traditional antibiotics: penicillin, methicillin, tetracycline, and erythromycin.

In 2005, at Georgetown University in Washington, D.C., researcher Dr Harry Preuss studied the lauric acid content of coconut oil. He found that it could inhibit the growth of many dangerous pathogenic microorganisms – including *Staph aureus*.

## Lauric Acid Prevents Fungal Infections Better than Prescription Drugs

Candida is another common infection that lauric acid found in coconut oil fights effectively. *Candidiasis* is a fungal infection that is responsible for yeast infections, athlete's foot, thrush, and even invasive candidiasis – where the bacterium enters the bloodstream.

The Department of Medical Microbiology & Parasitology, University College Hospital in Ibadan, Nigeria, studied the resistance of Candida to antibiotics and tested how coconut oil could be used to halt the growth of the fungus and prevent future outbreaks.

---

### ACNE PREVENTION: LAURIC ACID 15X STRONGER THAN BENZOYL PEROXIDE

Adult onset acne in your 30's and 40's is becoming a common occurrence for many men and women. Unfortunately, as skin ages, conventional acne treatments can prove to be too harsh and dehydrating to your skin.

The strong bactericidal properties of lauric acid were proven in a 2009 study from the University of California, Division of Dermatology. The study reviewed the antimicrobial efficacy of lauric acid against the bacteria *Propionibacterium acnes* (P. acnes), which causes inflammatory acne, and skin bacteria (*staph aureus* and *staph epidermis*), that aggravates existing acne.

Lauric acid tested 15 times more effective with stronger antimicrobial properties than that of benzoyl peroxide, proving that lauric acid is a potential alternative to traditional antibiotic treatment for acne.

In addition, the underlying factors of acne need to be addressed in treatment. Liver detoxification, maintaining healthy gut flora, increasing consumption of omega-3 fatty acids, and coconut oil taken internally can provide a **long-term natural solution** to acne.

---

17 different specimens of Candida were studied using coconut oil versus the antifungal drug fluconazole. The worse form, *Candida albicans*, was found to have the highest susceptibility to coconut oil as an antifungal agent.

Virgin coconut oil **proved to be more effective** than fluconazole, leading the researchers to state in their conclusion, "Coconut oil should be used in the treatment of drug-resistant evolving Candida species."

## Could Lauric Acid Treat HIV & Sexually Transmitted Diseases?

In 1987, the American Foundation for Aids Research (AMFAR) reviewed the antiviral lipid monolaurin as an alternative therapy for HIV. With antiviral drugs for HIV starting at $30,000 per year for treatment, an alternative food therapy option to assist in lowering the virus load would be extremely beneficial for HIV sufferers.

However, AMFAR did not pursue the research of lauric acid as a complementary treatment. Despite the fact that many pathogenic viruses and organisms – such as herpes simplex virus 1, measles virus, vesicular stomatitis virus, and visna virus – are destroyed by lauric acid.

When your body metabolizes lauric acid and capric acid in coconut oil, they're convert into monolaurin and monocaprin. These molecules have been shown to cause disintegration of HIV and the herpes virus. They destroy the fatty coating that surrounds herpes, HIV, and *Cytomegalovirus*.

A 1999 study by researchers from the University of Iceland, Reykjavik, recommended that a topical gel be developed with capric acid and lauric acid as active ingredients to be used for preventing sexually transmitted diseases such as herpes virus, secondary herpes fungal infections, HIV, gonorrhea, and Chlamydia.

Another potential benefit of using coconut oil is that it increases weight retention in late stage HIV patients who may have difficulty maintaining body weight.

## Monolaurin – the Missing Link in Your Diet

The coconut palm's name in Indian classics is 'Kalpavrisksha' or the "all-giving tree" and it's no wonder. The incredible benefits are abundantly clear.

Monolaurin cannot be produced by your body unless there is a source of lauric acid in your diet. Coconut oil is a rich source of lauric acid and can be used for treatment and disease prevention.

## Modern Day Disease Prevention with Coconut Oil

- ✓ The painful burning of a stomach ulcer can last for up to three hours. Coconut oil **kills the bacteria that leads to stomach ulcers** and can be used as a safe long-term remedy. Try consuming two to three tablespoons of virgin coconut oil daily as a preventative measure.

- ✓ Studies done by the Mayo Clinic in 1990 suggest that nearly all chronic cases of sinusitis are caused by fungi but are mistakenly mistreated with antibiotics. Chronic sinus infections are an immune system response to fungus. Coconut oil is antiviral and antifungal and can **help prevent sinus infections** before they start.

- ✓ Coconut oil has been proven to **kill microbes responsible for food poisoning**. Test animals were fed microbes, then coconut oil, and researchers noted that coconut oil killed the microbes.

- ✓ Another wonderful property of coconut oil is its ability to cleanse and **heal urinary tract infections (UTI)**. It only attacks harmful bacteria, leaving beneficial bacteria unharmed. To treat a UTI, take at least three tablespoons of virgin coconut oil every day. To encourage faster healing, drink two glasses of coconut water each day in addition to 8 glasses of purified water.

- ✓ With the nearly 50% lauric acid content of coconut oil, transformed into monolaurin by the body, **diarrhea doesn't stand a chance**. In the March 2010 *Journal of Ethnopharmacology*, researchers discovered that an extract taken from coconut oil was as effective as a leading anti-diarrhea medication. Try mixing ½ cup of shredded unsweetened coconut flakes with a tablespoon of coconut oil and roll into four to six balls. Eat one every hour or so until symptoms subside.

- ✓ Coconut oil is a **great insect repellant**. The active ingredient in most commercial insect repellants is 10% dodecanoic acid (DDA) that's been patented for this very reason. The active ingredient in DDA is a naturally occurring carboxylic acid *found in coconut oil* and is effective as a mosquito repellant.

- ✓ The polyphenol (antioxidant) capacity of coconut oil is a potent **parasite killing** substance. After 60 minutes, the parasite *Leishmania amazonensis* or sandfly, was killed.

- ✓ In traditional Mexican medicine, coconut oil has been used to **treat a sexually transmitted disease** known as trichomoniasis.

- ✓ Used as an **alternative to nonsteroidal anti-inflammatory drugs** (NSAIDs) – such as aspirin, ibuprofen, and naproxen – coconut oil has anti-inflammatory, analgesic, and fever-reducing properties without the side effects.

✓ The antiviral caprylic, capric, and lauric acids found in coconut oil accelerate your skin's ability for tissue regeneration and act as a **protective barrier against pressure ulcers and bedsores**.

## Lauric Acid in Coconut Oil Proven to Heal Wounds and Burns

On the eastern Indonesian island of Flores, the Ngada people have a rich history of using coconut oil, along with medicinal plants such as papaya and betel nut, to treat wounds. The short carbon structure of lauric acid in coconut oil prevents it from becoming rancid in tropical climates, making it ideal for wound treatment.

A fascinating study by the Department of Biochemistry, University of Kerala, India evaluated the effectiveness of coconut oil on open wounds for 14 days. They reviewed skin regrowth, collagen levels, and tissue healing patterns.

Wounds treated with virgin coconut oil healed much faster and developed a higher cell turnover of collagen than untreated wounds.

Even the antioxidant enzyme activity of glutathione – an extremely important anti-aging molecule called the "mother of all antioxidants" – tested at increased levels by the 10th day of treating wounds with coconut oil.

A unique burn wound healing treatment studied by the Department of Pharmacology, KMC International Centre in Manipal, India found that silver sulphadiazine (also known as Silvadene) when combined with virgin coconut oil aided in faster healing.

This combination even reduced scarring and decreased risk of infection by a significant percentage. Coconut oil is an effective burn wound healing agent. New blood vessels form more quickly in skin treated with virgin coconut oil. This also aids the body in producing healthy skin that is free of scarring.

**The wound healing process goes through three critical phases.**

Inflammatory Phase**:**

Your wound starts to clot or stops oozing fluid and/or pus. White blood cells gather and your body begins the process of forming new collagen. This phase typically lasts two to seven days.

It's important to keep your wound clean. Coat liberally with coconut oil several times a day at this stage to stimulate collagen formation.

Proliferative Phase**:**

In this phase, your body is producing new capillaries and knitting together the wound. New cells are being formed which causes the wound to have a "wet" look.

Your body continues to produce collagen, so it's important to take at least two to three tablespoons of coconut oil daily to assist in the healing process. I recommend you build up your tolerance to coconut oil by starting with one tablespoon a day and gradually increasing your dosage.

Apply coconut oil topically to the wound two to three times a day with a clean swab or gauze pad.

Maturation Phase:

This is final stage of scar tissue healing. Your body produces more collagen and slowly forms the scar so the excess collagen is reabsorbed and the scar becomes less visible. It could take almost two years for scars to reach their final appearance.

Apply coconut oil topically by massaging the scar several times daily once fully healed. This will help your body break down scar tissue and keep it from becoming stiff.

**Nature's Gift**

The healing gift of coconut oil is one that keeps on giving. There is so much more to be discovered.

You will find out how coconut oil and other powerful healing fats can help you build a better body, by protecting your brain, guarding your heart, strengthening your bones, boosting your antioxidant capacity, transforming your oral health, and balancing your hormones.

CHAPTER 5

# THE FAT-FUELED BULLETPROOF BRAIN

## Protect AND Repair Your Brain with Ketone Bodies

There are over 36.5 million cases of dementia around the world and the number of diagnosed cases is projected to double every 20 years.

---

She sensed something was wrong. Her thoughts seemed to vanish into a deep fog. She looked at a face and although she knew who he was, she could not remember his name. She would start a conversation with someone and then mid-sentence she would forget the entire discussion.

Her job was high pressure and it meant everything to her. Her increasing forgetfulness made it difficult to maintain her performance. She struggled for two years before deciding it was time to take a break. After a much-needed vacation, she returned to work invigorated and renewed, but something still wasn't right.

She decided it was time to see a doctor. At only 51 years old, she was diagnosed with the beginning stages of Alzheimer's disease, a common form of dementia. With no family history of the disease and in great health, she was devastated.

This is the true account of Patti Smith, a corporate banker, as reported by Dr. Bruce Fife of the *Coconut Research Center*.

---

Alzheimer's disease (AD) is terrifying. In the United States, it is second only to cancer as the most feared health condition. Most cases are diagnosed in people over the age of 60, but for some – like Patti Smith – it can begin as early as the 40s. Nearly 2.5 million people will be diagnosed with early-onset Alzheimer's like Patti.

Women are at the center of the Alzheimer's epidemic. 1-in-6 females are at risk for developing the disease.

Right now, there is no cure.

The earliest symptoms can be easy to dismiss...confusion and mild forgetfulness. The progression of AD is different for every case – while some may gradually worsen, others can experience a much faster deterioration. Over time, brain function becomes impaired to the point that it cannot be ignored and becomes obvious to the people around you.

- Difficulty organizing thoughts
- Repetitive statements and questions
- Forgetting recent conversations or events
- Consistently losing track of belongings
- Inability to recall familiar names and places
- Loss of time and days
- Deterioration of reading, writing, and speaking skills
- Lack of concentration
- Basic tasks are unfamiliar or confusing
- Changes to moods and behavior that can include anxiety, distrust, and depression

Losing the memories of who you are and the people who have been part of your life can make those with AD feel trapped in a prison of their own mind. Recent memories are the first to go and as the disease progresses, more years are swallowed up in the abyss. Childhood memories and learned information are the last to be robbed from the mind of a patient with Alzheimer's disease, leaving them helpless and confused.

It is agonizing for the AD patient and for those friends and family who are slowly *erased* from the mind of the person they love.

However, there are ways to **prevent and reverse** Alzheimer's disease. The secret lies in the healing power of coconut oil's ketones.

According to neurologist Dr. David Perlmutter, author of *Grain Brain*, it is the flawed U.S. nutritional food pyramid (11 servings of grain daily), the over-consumption of wheat, and the removal of fat in American diets that are the root cause of the Alzheimer's pandemic.

Recent studies have uncovered that both **fat and cholesterol are severely deficient** in the Alzheimer's brain. Both fat and cholesterol are crucial brain nutrients.

The brain represents only 2% of the body's total mass but utilizes 25% of the total cholesterol. Cholesterol and fat are essential to transmit nerve signals and fight off infections.

The core cause of the effects of Alzheimer's is the brain's inability to process the primary fuel of blood sugar or glucose to produce energy. As a result, the brain is deprived of the energy it requires to repair brain cells and stimulate the growth of new cells.

Glucose is the primary source of energy and if your brain can't process it, an alternative fuel is needed or the cells begin to atrophy.

Ketones are a special type of high-energy fuel created by the liver when the body burns through its fat stores. When glucose levels drop, the body steps in and increases ketone production as an alternative to glucose. The problem is that ketone production only increases when carbohydrate intake is very low.

If you switch to consuming primarily proteins and fats, then your body can produce all the nutrients needed from ketones. This type of diet is known as a ketogenic diet (such as South Beach Diet and other similar eating plans). However, total daily carbohydrate intake must remain at or below 2% for it to work. That means over 90% of your calories need to come from fat.

Studies from The John M. Freeman Pediatric Epilepsy Center, Johns Hopkins Hospital, Baltimore, Maryland published in 2006 on the neuroprotective and disease-modifying effects of the ketogenic diet have rocked the medical community. Researchers raised the possibility that the ketogenic diet could be disease transforming for those suffering from Alzheimer's.

Ketogenic diets have been effectively used to treat epilepsy for over 90 years. Using it to treat other diseases isn't a long reach.

On the other hand, making a complete meal out of solid lard or butter doesn't sound appealing...and how much meat can a human eat before crying "uncle?"

## Coconut Ketones Unlock the Key to Reversing Alzheimer's

The saturated fat in coconut oil is composed of 65% medium-chain triglycerides (MCTs). What makes MCTs so special is that when they are ingested, they are rapidly absorbed and converted into ketones regardless of blood glucose levels or the amount carbohydrates present in the diet.

**Simply stated, coconut oil provides ketone bodies for fuel that the brain can use quickly no matter what the rest of your diet looks like!**

---

A trailblazing study in 2004 from the journal *Neurobiology of Aging* found that the administration of medium-chain triglycerides (MCTs), the primary fat in coconut oil, almost instantly improved cognitive performance in older adults suffering from memory loss, dementia, and even Alzheimer's. The improvement didn't happen after weeks or months of treatment, but after **a single 40 ml dose** (about 3 US tablespoons)!

---

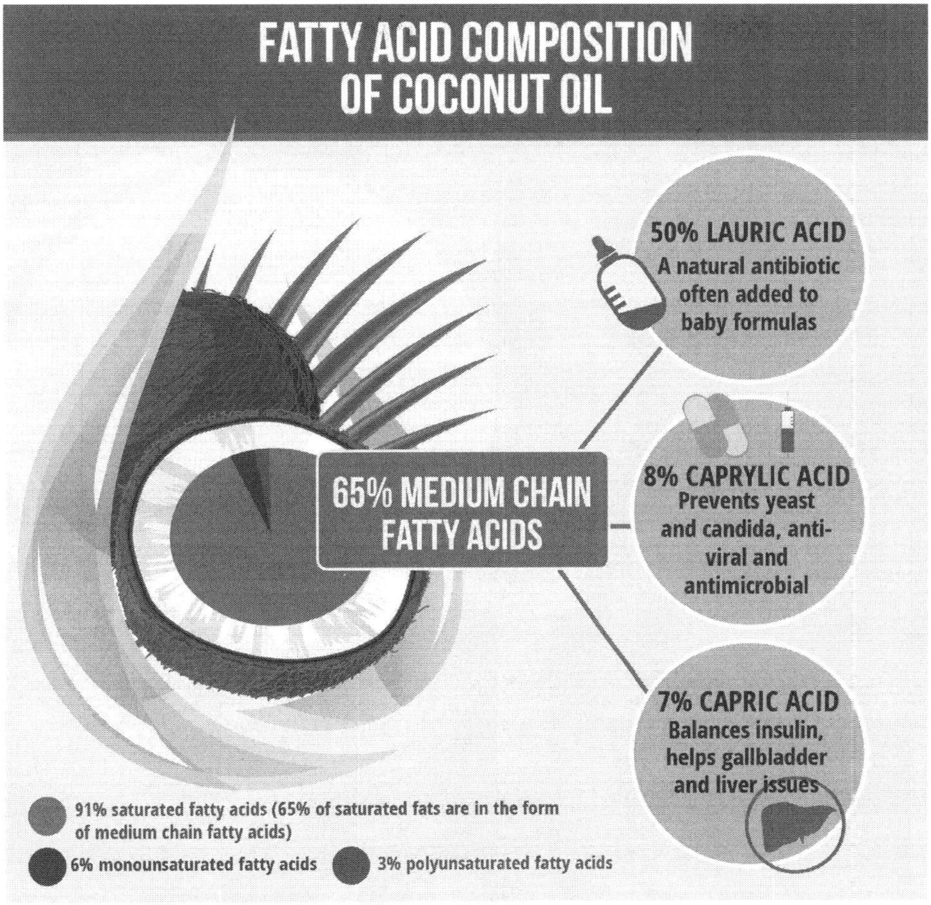


Almost 20 subjects with diagnosed Alzheimer's disease or other forms of mild cognitive impairment were given either emulsified MCTs or a placebo. The researchers noted a significant increase in blood plasma levels of the ketone body beta-Hydroxybutyric acid (beta-OHB) **after only 90 minutes of treatment**.

Studies in neurobiological science advise that ketone bodies such as beta-OHB are indeed an effective and more efficient energy alternative for the brain when blood glucose is low.

This energy is needed for nerve cell survival and for synaptic activity, which is the basis of learning and memory.

*MCTS (or medium chain fatty acids MCFA) are more rapidly absorbed by the body and more quickly burned as fuel instead of LCFA (long chain fatty acids) and stored as fat. Coconut oil ketone bodies are a very simple alternative to glucose that the body can use for fuel. The liver metabolizes ketone bodies immediately and your brain can immediately use it for fuel.*

In patent applications for MCT oil (a derivative of coconut oil) over 47% of participants tested showed remarkable improvement in their cognitive (memory) scores after just one dose!

To get the maximum benefit of the healing powers of coconut oil, I recommend using virgin coconut oil rather than MCT oil. MCT oil is missing the important immune boosting component of monolaurin (lauric acid) found in natural virgin coconut oil.

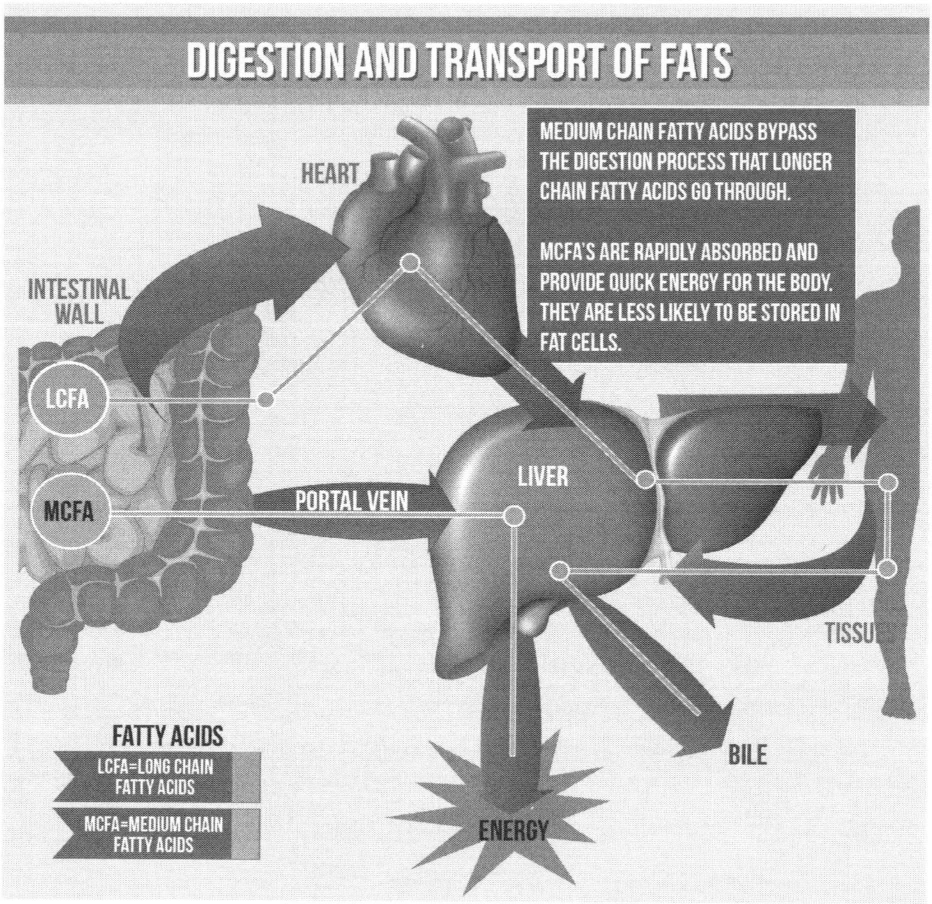

# MARY NEWPORT, MD OVERCOMES ALZHEIMER'S WITH COCONUT OIL

**A Remarkable True Story**

Dr. Mary Newport is the person who created the term "coconut ketones" through her own remarkable experience. She uses it to describe how she personally used virgin coconut oil – available everywhere these days – to boost ketone levels in the blood without extreme fasting or a diet that removes all carbohydrates.

When your body is in "starvation" mode or restricted from carbs, your liver kicks into gear making ketones so that your brain can be fed and you can keep functioning.

With coconut oil, neither of those scenarios is necessary.

Her fight to beat back the devastating effects of Alzheimer's disease began with her husband of more than thirty years. Steve Newport started showing signs of forgetfulness, which rapidly deteriorated until he was diagnosed in 2003 with early-onset Alzheimer's disease in his early fifties.

After the shock and horror of his diagnosis wore off, they spent years trying to find drug trials and alternative treatments that would preserve his quality of life.

Mary, a successful doctor who ran a pediatric intensive care unit at a Florida hospital, tried traditional treatments but they didn't help and Steve's condition continued to worsen. He could no longer read, could not do simple math (he'd been an accountant by trade), and the aggressive nature of his particular case made him ineligible for clinical trials.

She discovered that one drug being researched for an Alzheimer's treatment contained medium-chain triglycerides (MCTs) as its primary ingredient. Initial research looked good but there wasn't even a clinical trial in the works for the potential treatment yet. After being denied participation in another trial, Mary became desperate.

With nothing to lose, no potential side effects, and a husband she desperately wanted to help, she began to use a readily available, natural source of MCT – coconut oil.

The results have fascinated Steve's doctors. Coconut oil dramatically slowed the progression of atrophy in Steve's brain. In fact, his scores in cognitive testing drastically improved. It is a result that was unheard of before his case. Alzheimer's disease steals cognitive function and never gives it back.

Over the next two years, Steve continued to improve.

In a recent update, Mary told an interviewer that Steve has experienced setbacks in the six years since he began taking coconut oil – such as the emotional trauma of losing his father and a fall that resulted in a head injury.

She said that the disease remains, it has not been cured, but she credits coconut oil with having him with her – in relatively good health and still recognizing her as his beloved wife.

Steve's Alzheimer's case was incredibly aggressive. His cognitive function was deteriorating rapidly before Mary tried treatment with coconut oil. Without coconut oil, she states adamantly, she would have lost her husband years ago. *Alzheimer's Disease: What If There Was a Cure? By Mary T. Newport, M.D., excerpt from the Coconut Research Center*

---

**Insights on Steve Newport's Case**

There are those who focus on the fact that Steve Newport still has Alzheimer's disease rather than the fact that he gained much of his life back when his doctors believed that all hope was lost. Naysayers mention that "not everyone" has had the same results with their own loved ones and that it is wrong to "dash the hopes" of those struggling with AD.

*Perhaps they're right...*

There is no cure for Alzheimer's and perhaps Steve's treatment will not work in every case (as is the fact with any method of treatment). However, coconut oil is healthy, well tolerated, and has no side effects. If even one patient is helped by this harmless and inexpensive treatment – is that not worth it?

Traditional drugs did not help Steve. His condition was declining rapidly. If coconut oil gave him two solid years that he would not have had otherwise – should Mary Newport regret those years simply because her husband isn't "cured?"

When Mary's husband became a victim of this awful neurodegenerative disease, she tried everything and finally thought, "What is there to lose?"

She lost *nothing* and Steve gained several years of being "present" in his own life. There is no doubt in my own mind that this couple definitely found their investment in coconut oil "worth it."

## Anti-Inflammatory Effects of Coconut Oil on the Brain

Inflammation or free radical production is what causes much of the damage in the brains of Alzheimer's and dementia patients. In fact, inflammation has been linked to so many serious diseases at this point in the medical community – by researchers all over the world – that it is *shocking* there isn't more outcry from the general population on what causes it and how to stop it.

What causes inflammation?

Sugar – It's everywhere, it may be hidden in the labels, but look closely at the foods you eat and you'll find cane sugar, agave nectar, crystalline fructose, and high fructose corn syrup. It may be sugar by a different name but *it is still sugar.*

Sugar sets you on a roller coaster of emotions, plays chaos with your energy levels, and changes your immune system, hormones, and gut. Most importantly, it alters your cell membranes and creates the ideal environment for total body inflammation.

Food intolerances – Gluten (wheat), soy, and corn are highly allergenic foods. With hybridization, these three crops are the most genetically modified foods (GMOs) on the planet. It's no wonder that your immune system can't recognize them. Once digested, these foods can create inflammation in your brain and immune system that sets off chain reactions in every cell.

Try a simple diet overhaul.

Eat grass-fed meats, wild fish, eggs, fruits, tree nuts, and vegetables. Stay away from corn, legumes, soy, processed diary, and grains for 30 days. Choose organic whenever you can.

In addition, **every day** add at least two tablespoons of virgin coconut oil to your diet.

You will give your brain the extra fuel it needs to restore the balance and nutrients that it's been starved of…think of it as a jumpstart for your brain. Within a few days, you'll notice clarity and energy you've probably been lacking for years.

**Two powerful antioxidant compounds found in coconut oil,** ferulic acid and p-coumaric acid**, help reduce and reverse the effects of inflammation.**

Ferulic acid – A polyphenol found in the cell walls of tomatoes and rice bran, the name is Greek and means "the one that does not wither." It scavenges and destroys several different types of free radicals and reactive nitrogen species (RNS) that create inflammation of the brain and neuronal dysfunction. Ferulic acid also prevents cell death, which slows down the aging process.

p-Coumaric acid – Found in honey, vinegar, and wine, p-coumaric increases immune system response, lowers plaque build-up in artery walls, and decreases LDL (bad) cholesterol levels.

Together these two compounds have a synergistic effect. They are responsible for over **80% of the potent antioxidant power** of coconut oil.

Add coconut oil to your diet. Evaluate how you feel, listen to your body, and make your own judgment call about this healing fat of life.

## How Thyroid Imbalance Increases Your Risk of Alzheimer's Disease

Another often-overlooked factor in the loss of cognitive functions is problems with your thyroid hormones. Thyroid hormones are essential for brain development, energy and metabolism, skin, muscles, and your heart. An imbalance in hormones can cause your body functions to swing wildly out of control

Hypothyroidism (underactive thyroid) is most commonly caused by inflammation, certain autoimmune disorders (Hashimoto's disease), viral and bacterial infections, diet, and as a side effect of radiation cancer treatment.

It has been directly linked to personality and behavior conditions (bipolar disorders, depression, dementia, and personality disorders), weight gain, changes in skin and hair, irregular heartbeat, and fatigue. Even short-term thyroid hormone deficiency can create lasting brain damage and structural brain defects.

Hyperthyroidism (overactive thyroid) can be caused by certain autoimmune diseases (such as Graves), diet, or when your thyroid experiences inflammation from another source.

It can lead to unexplained weight loss, anxiety, changes to the menstrual cycle, irregular heartbeat, muscle weakness, changes in skin and hair, and mild to severe mood swings.

Polyunsaturated oils block thyroid hormone secretion. They also wreak havoc on your cells and create free radical damage. You should avoid these oils as they have been proven to disrupt thyroid function, which contributes to Alzheimer's disease.

- Vegetable oil
- Soybean oil

- Canola or Rapeseed oil
- Corn oil
- Sunflower oil
- Grapeseed oil
- Safflower oil
- Rice Bran oil

**Coconut oil supports thyroid function and thyroid governs brain development**, including the production of new myelin sheaths (essential for a proper functioning nervous system). The key role that coconut oil plays in protecting your brain from Alzheimer's disease is clear.

- Tips for Prevention**:** Take two to four tablespoons of coconut oil daily for coconut ketone fuel.
- Avoid refined fructose and sugar that lead to inflammation and "type 3 diabetes" – one term many doctors are giving Alzheimer's disease.
- Avoid wheat – the blood brain barrier is negatively affected by gluten, which promotes inflammation and autoimmunity that can lead to the development of dementia and Alzheimer's disease.
- Keep your gut flora healthy with a daily probiotic and fermented foods.
- Avoid aluminum found in antiperspirants, non-stick cookware, and even some vaccines.
- Avoid statin drugs (found most commonly in antidepressants, cholesterol medications, and pain relievers), which contain compounds that block a nervous system transmitter called acetylcholine and have been shown to increase your risk of dementia.

## How Much Coconut Oil Should You Take to Protect Your Memory and Prevent Cognitive Decline?

Therapeutic levels of MCTs have been studied at 1.5 tablespoons (20 grams) per day. Try starting with two tablespoons of coconut oil (30 grams) daily as a preventative measure. It can be added to your coffee or tea, blended in a green smoothie, or used in meal preparation.

For treatment purposes, a total of 5 tablespoons (75 grams) of coconut oil a day taken with meals is recommended. It's best to consult with your doctor or health practitioner, especially for treatment purposes since each person's case is unique.

You can add a portion of the coconut oil to each of the three meals you consume during the day. It takes approximately three hours for your body to process the coconut oil and the benefits to begin to take effect.

There are **no side effects of coconut oil** as long as you are not allergic to coconuts.

However, give your body a chance to adjust by starting slowly and building up your consumption. If you start too quickly with too much, some people report "loose" bowels, nausea, or a bit of gas.

Starting with a single tablespoon every day will get you on the right track!

Take back control of what you put in your body to help heal your mind and experience the difference it will make in your clarity, mood, memory, and overall cognition.

## Coconut Oil and Turmeric – A Dynamic Alzheimer's and Depression Fighting Duo

Turmeric's bright orange-yellow color and mild taste are easy to overlook. You probably know it best as the spice that gives curried dishes around the world its unique color and flavor.

Nevertheless, this Eastern spice has a proven place in the scientific community after years of research.

The star of the ginger family, turmeric is naturally anti-inflammatory, antioxidant, neuroprotective, and neurochemical. All due to its active compound **curcumin**.

This powerful antioxidant has been the source of heavy research over the last decade. Scientists have discovered that curcumin can help ease Alzheimer's symptoms caused by oxidation and inflammation and is effective as a natural way to fight depression.

A recent 2014 study by the Department of Pharmacology, Government Medical College, in Guajart, India conducted a six-week trial on 60 patients diagnosed with major depressive disorder. The test participants were divided into three groups and randomized.

- Prozac only
- Prozac plus 1gram of oil-based curcumin
- Curcumin only

The most effective treatment was found to be group two (77.8%), followed by Prozac (64.7%), then Curcumin (62.5%). It is fascinating that curcumin fell within less than 3% effectiveness of the dangerous pharmaceutical drug but the results didn't take into account the "active placebo" effect.

Dr. Irving Kirsch documented that patients treated with antidepressants respond to the expectations around the treatment "it's working!" rather than to the medication itself.

The conclusion of the study provides the first real clinical evidence that curcumin may be used an effective and safe modality for treatment in patients with major depressive disorder. It could prove to be a useful alternative for those patients with severe depression that do not respond to antidepressants.

The authors of the study emphasized curcumin's high degree of safety up to dosages of 12g daily. In addition, it wasn't specified what type of oil was used in the study...it could have been corn or soy oil!

Can you imagine the powerful brain-boosting properties of coconut oil, when combined with the potent Neuroprotective antioxidant capabilities of turmeric? Such a safe and simple way to protect your memory, fight Alzheimer's, and even prevent depression!

Turmeric – when added to coconut oil – supports glutathione synthesis, which prevents inflammation, helps regulate hormones, increases the production of neurotransmitters, and encourages brain cell regeneration.

When cooking with turmeric, always mix it with coconut oil and use freshly ground black pepper as the oil and the pepper help increase absorption.

Do your best to sneak 1 tablespoon of turmeric into your meals every day. Try it in scrambled eggs or add 2 tablespoons to tomato sauce over roasted eggplant or zucchini for a vibrant flavor you're going to love.

# CHAPTER 6
# HEART HEALTHY FAT WISE: THE TRIFECTA OF HEALING FATS

Gary Taubes published an article in the *New York Times* back in 2002 called "What If It's all Been a Big Fat Lie?" His essay pointed to the findings of Walter Willet, chairman of the Department of Nutrition at the Harvard School of Public Health.

Willet ran a comprehensive study on 300,000 individuals (that cost over $100 million dollars) that contradicted the findings of the "low-fat is good" message back in the 1980s.

At the height of the low-fat dogma, the obesity epidemic was climbing, heart disease still ruled as the number one silent killer, and type 2 diabetes rose steadily. All due to the fact the percentage of fat consumed had drastically decreased in the American diet for the prior twenty years.

Willet pointed out that if Americans were eating less fat and fat was the cause behind heart disease and skyrocketing cholesterol levels, then we should be seeing fewer incidents of heart disease instead of it affecting 1-in-4 adults in the United States.

In his interview with Taubes, Willet said, "That is very disconcerting; it suggests that something else bad is happening."

*Nearly 600,000 people die of heart disease in the United States every year.*

Where are all the good things that were supposed to happen when people were told to cut "evil, death-causing fat" out of their diets? Where are the health benefits to removing fat? Where is the evidence that less fat has made us a healthier nation?

Heart Disease is the #1 Silent Killer:

- 25 % of adults in the United States takes statins
- 75 million Americans suffer from heart disease
- 20 million have diabetes
- 57 million have pre-diabetes

In March of 2013, the World Health Organization (WHO) published that 30% of all global deaths – **17.3 million people** – was a direct result of cardiovascular diseases. The future doesn't look any better. WHO predicted that this number would reach **23.3 million people** by the year 2030. Such a date seems like the distant future but it is a mere 15 years away.

Fat supposedly causes heart disease but we're losing more than 17 million people every year despite efforts to remove it from our diet. Something doesn't add up.

## Why Sugar and Starch Are Deadly for Your Heart

Heart surgeon Dr. Dwight Lundell published a confessional essay on "What Really Causes Heart Disease" that went viral. Ultimately, it appeared on over 237,000 Facebook walls.

Here's an excerpt of that article:

---

> I freely admit to being wrong. As a heart surgeon with 25 years' experience, having performed over 5,000 open-heart surgeries, today is my day to right the wrong with medical and scientific fact.
>
> We opinion makers insisted heart disease resulted from the simple fact of elevated blood cholesterol. The only accepted therapy was prescribing medications to lower cholesterol and a diet that severely restricted fat intake. The latter of course we insisted would lower cholesterol and heart disease. Deviations from these recommendations were considered heresy and could quite possibly result in malpractice.
>
> *The real culprit behind heart disease isn't fat, it's inflammation.*
>
> The injury and inflammation in our blood vessels is caused by the low fat diet recommended for years by mainstream medicine.
>
> What are the biggest culprits of chronic inflammation? Quite simply, they are the overload of simple, highly processed carbohydrates (sugar, flour, and all the products made from them) and the excess consumption of omega-6 vegetable oils like soybean, corn, and sunflower that are found in many processed foods.

---

You can probably understand the ripple effect of shock this sent through the medical community!

Cinnamon rolls, processed breads, cakes, and industrial baked goods that are packed with sugar and simple carbohydrates, processed omega-6 oils, have been abundant in the American diet for the past sixty years. These kinds of foods have been slowly poisoning all of us.

Your consumption of omega-6 oils should be at a 1:1 ratio with omega-3 oils.

Not so in the average Western diet! The typical ratio is between 15:1 to as high as 30:1 in favor of omega-6. Too many omega-6 oils in the diet cause your cell membranes to create a chemical called cytokines.

**Cytokines directly cause inflammation.**

If a food contains corn, soy, canola, safflower, or sunflower oil...those are omega-6 oils and they are destroying your body from the inside out. You want to avoid them at all costs!

Along with omega-6 oils, sugars and starches create even more inflammation. When you eat a delicious doughnut, your body responds instantly, sounding an alarm as if an intruder has arrived.

Your pancreas secretes insulin, which drives sugar into each cell, where it is stored as energy.

When your cells are full and reject the extra glucose, blood sugar rises, producing more insulin, and glucose converts to stored fat.

How does glucose create heart disease?

Blood sugar is tightly controlled by the body. Extra glucose molecules attach to various proteins that rough up the blood vessel wall, much like sandpaper on wood. This repeated injury creates inflammation in your blood vessels.

You end up with fat cells that create huge quantities of pro-inflammatory chemicals.

Dr. Lunden continues, "The process that began with a sweet roll turns into a vicious cycle over time that creates heart disease, high blood pressure, diabetes, and finally, Alzheimer's disease, as the inflammatory process continues unabated."

Choosing healthy healing fats and sticking to carbohydrates found in colorful fruits and vegetables, you'll add years to your life and reverse the damage caused by the standard Western diet.

## Is A Steak Really A Heart Attack on a Plate?

Animal fats in particular contain less than 20% omega-6 and are less likely to cause inflammation. Cholesterol isn't the cause of heart disease.

From the early 1970s, meat consumption was shunned in favor of more grains and low-fat diets. A juicy steak was considered a "heart attack on a plate" and associated with coronary heart disease, strokes, and even diabetes.

Was meat really to blame?

The Harvard School of Public Health, Department of Epidemiology in Boston, Massachusetts compiled a meta-analysis of 1,218,380 individuals. Of these cases, 23,889 had coronary heart disease, 2280 were victims of stroke, and 10,797 were diabetics.

All data was pooled and it was discovered that red meat intake was not associated with coronary heart disease. However, *processed meat* intake (such as hot dogs and lunchmeat) was associated with a 42% higher risk of coronary heart disease and diabetes.

Always select organic grass-fed beef, buffalo, bison, lamb, and pasture-raised pigs and chickens. Organic means that no antibiotics, hormones, or pesticides were used in raising the animal. Simply choosing "grass-fed" and "pasture-raised" means that animals are not being raised in confined animal feeding operations (CAFO).

Cattle raised in such environments results in food that is unhealthy for humans with greater risk of contamination and disease among animals crammed in close quarters. Not to mention what they're fed and injected with during their lifetime.

**How the Healing Fat Butter Won the War against the Low-Fat Brigade**

*Time Magazine* admitted in their groundbreaking cover story of 2014 that they were wrong about vilifying saturated fats.

In their searing exposé, they uncover the junk science behind the claims that saturated fat was the enemy. You would think that such a well-respected magazine blowing the lid off the fat lie would start a chain reaction of scientific fact, a change in direction of what the food manufacturers and media have been telling us for decades.

Not so much.

Mainstream media won't admit defeat and reversing decades of bad press is not an easy task.

Don't expect the giant food manufacturers to switch to real saturated fats in their products.

In fact, one of the world's largest margarine producers admitted that they had been wrong about butter from the beginning. What's their solution? They decided to add some of the "real" stuff into their trans-fat yellow fake "food." You would be shocked to know that before margarine is colored it is a stomach-turning shade of gray.

What's even more disturbing is that their little bit of "real" butter will come from milk treated with hormones, antibiotics, fed GMO feed, and produced in confined animal feeding operations.

Butter quality is determined by its fat content, freshness, and salt levels. Salt preserves butter, so "salted butter" has a longer shelf life. For butter manufacturers, salted butter means they can sell you an older product. For you, since you don't know what type of salt was used, it can also mean there are probably hidden chemicals in your butter.

There are incredible benefits to choosing grass-fed butter – even more than simple "organic" butter. Grass-fed butter means the cows have grazed on green grass instead of traditional grain feed that is likely tainted with GMOs.

Grass-fed butter is darker in color and has a richer, more complex taste than the normal sweet creaminess of organic butter. In addition, pasture or grass-fed butter has a better nutrient profile and is considered a heart-healthy superfood.

### Nutrient Profile of Grass-Fed Butter

- Conjugated Linoleic Acid (CLA) reduces cardiovascular disease, lowers cholesterol, protects against cancer, and helps your body build muscle
- Omega-3 fatty acids protect cardiovascular function and contains arachidonic acid which is vital for brain function and skin health are both found in grass-fed butter
- Packed with vitamins A, E, and K2 for optimal heart health.
- Contains the essential minerals manganese, chromium, zinc, copper, and selenium
- Iodine that you require for thyroid health

Grass-fed butter even reduces inflammation. This is crucial, since internal inflammation is where heart disease has now been proven to begin. The natural compounds in grass-fed butter contain the sort of cholesterol that is vital for your heart, brain, and nervous system. There are also various natural compounds with anti-fungal and even anti-cancer properties. It also raises HDL (good) cholesterol, which is associated with a lower risk of heart disease.

## Grass-Fed Butter and Vitamin K2 – The Most Important Nutrient to Prevent a Heart Attack

If you mention vitamin K, you'll probably get quizzical looks since most people don't know about it. It is hands down the most important nutrient for your heart.

Vitamin K1 is found in dark leafy greens and vitamin K2 is found in high-fat dairy products produced from grass-fed cows, egg yolks, liver, and natto (fermented soybeans).

Vitamin K2 helps to keep your arteries clear and calcium-free. Artery calcification occurs when blood vessels or valvular tissue becomes mineralized. Calcium deposits leach out from the bones, into the arteries, and this is the start of atherosclerotic (hardening of the arteries) vascular disease.

The Rotterdam Study was established in the Netherlands in 1990 and focused on the population-wide causes of cardiovascular disease (among others) in the elderly residents of their country. The study continued for two decades and is considered one of the most comprehensive scientific projects in recent history.

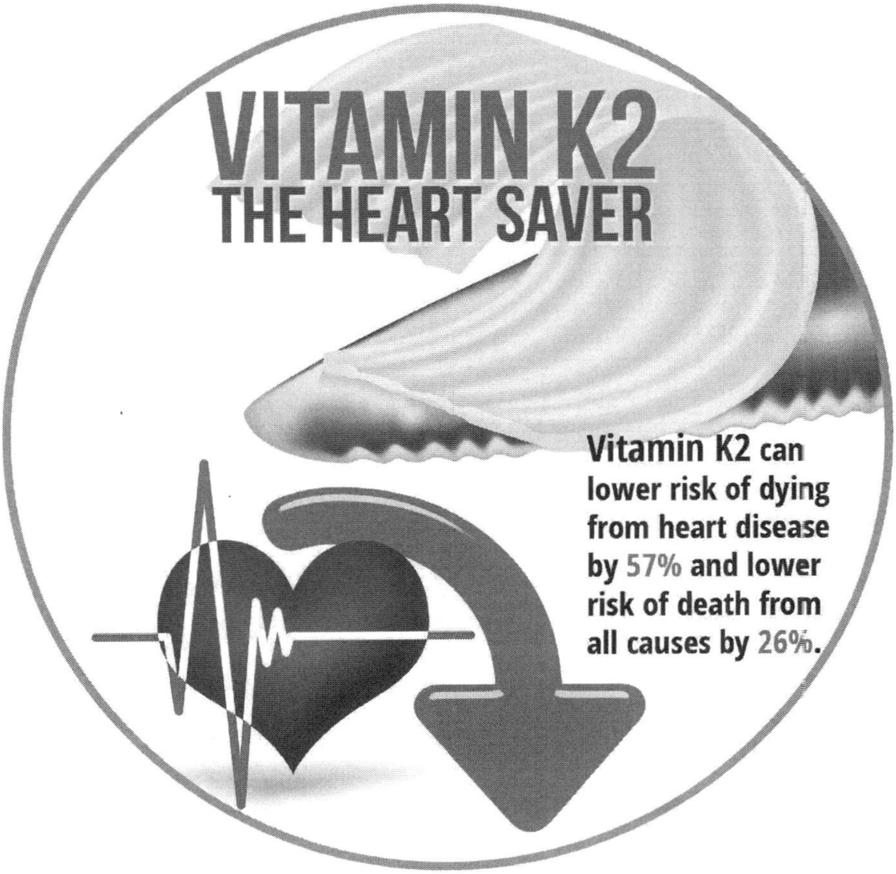


Researchers particularly examined the effects of vitamin K2 on heart disease. Participants who had the highest intake had a **57% lower risk of dying from heart disease** and a **26% lower risk of death** from all causes.

The advice of the low-fat mainstream health practitioners and government nutritionists was sadly wrong and created the pandemic of heart disease that we are dealing with today.

Every bite you consume must come from natural REAL WHOLE food. The margarine manufacturers – just as all the companies making cheap, fake food – are betting that you won't spend more on real butter versus the fake stuff.

It's up to you and me to prove them wrong.

## Animal Fat vs. Safflower Oil

A sample of 458 middle-aged Australian men (30-59) took part in the Sydney Diet Heart Study. The participants had experienced a heart attack or suffered from angina (chest pain). Half were advised to cut their animal fat intake and replace it with safflower oil (similar to sunflower oil) and safflower oil margarine. They were also given safflower oil supplements to take.

The other half continued to consume their normal diet that contained animal fat. What were the results? The men who ate more of the safflower-derived products were almost **twice as likely to die from all causes** including heart disease!

Saturated fats – found in grass-fed butter, coconut oil, and animal meats – have already been identified as key components of your cell membranes, essential for the production of hormones, and the absorption of vitamins and minerals.

You cannot survive without them.

## Vitamin-Packed Healing Fat: Red Palm Oil

Now that the tide is turning on the once-perceived link between dietary fats and cardiovascular disease, new interest has been sparked in the ancient antioxidant-rich red palm oil.

Red palm oil dates back more than 5,000 years and was so highly valued by pharaohs in ancient Egypt that they had it placed in their tombs upon death.

The bright orange-red fruit derives it color from carotenes (also found in tomatoes and carrots). Red palm oil is not to be confused with palm kernel oil. Red palm oil or palm oil is composed of approximately 50% saturated fatty acids, 40% monounsaturated fatty acids, and 10% polyunsaturated fatty acids.

The Oxidative Stress Research Centre, Department of Biomedical Sciences, Cape Peninsula University, in Bellville, South Africa, studied red palm oil and determined that it does not promote atherosclerosis (hardening of the arteries) or arterial thrombosis (blood clots in vessels).

In fact, red palm oil protects against heart disease, destroys free radicals, reduces oxidative stress, and lowers blood pressure. When consumed in moderation, it helps with nutrient absorption, activates red blood cell production, and even improves immune function. Red palm oil contains a high concentration of antioxidants that reduce LDL (bad) cholesterol levels.

- Beta-carotene (vitamin A)
- Tocotrienols (which contain **60 times** the antioxidant activity of ordinary vitamin E and strengthen the heart so it can withstand stress)
- Tocopherols
- Vitamin E
- Lycopene
- Vitamin K
- CoQ10

Red palm oil is an excellent cooking oil for baking, sautéing, and med um-heat frying. It remains stable up to 302 degrees F.

When purchasing red palm oil, always look for **organic unrefined** oil, since many available on the market are non-organic and sprayed with harsh chemical herbicides. Some red palm oils may have a harsh taste, but look for those that are **cold-pressed** or **cold-filtered**. This type of processing will give you a mild carrot-like flavor and buttery texture. Always check if the red palm oil you are purchasing has been sustainably harvested to ensure that no deforestation or animal habitat destruction has taken place.

## The Healing Fat Virgin Coconut Oil and Your Heart

The diseased heart is an energy-deficient heart. If you improve oxygen flow and fuel delivery – survival is dramatically improved.

Virgin coconut oil contains medium-chain fatty acids (MCFAs) that have distinct physical and metabolic properties that make them a readily available energy source, particularly among those with cardiomyopathy (heart muscle disease).

Since the medium-chain fatty acids in coconut oil are a smaller particle size, it makes a huge difference in how it is processed by your body.

MCFAs are metabolized in a unique way. They do not require pancreatic digestive enzymes or bile so they put little strain on the body's digestive system.

MCFAs are preferred by the heart to use as fuel instead of glucose or polyunsaturated fatty acids. Ketones, which are produced from MCFAs, act as a super fuel for the heart because they increase oxygen delivery by 39% and heart function by 28%.

Once they pass through the stomach, they are efficiently utilized by the body and do not circulate in the bloodstream like other fats. In fact, coconut oil MCFAs are used by the body to produce energy rather than store fat. These unique properties of MCFAs have been used for more than 50 years for treating lipid (fat) absorption disorders.

The Université François Rabelais, in Tours, France confirmed in their research that coconut oil is not harmful to the heart and listed many of its therapeutic uses.

This is reinforced by examining the Polynesian people of Pukapuka and Tokelau. Both populations eat high quantities of saturated fat from coconuts – 63% and 34% of their diet, respectively. Yet vascular disease is uncommon in either society. There's no evidence that high saturated fat intake is harmful to the citizenry of these small nations.

Coconut oil may slightly increase total cholesterol levels but this is due to the increase in HDL (good) cholesterol. Researchers at Harvard Medical School found that even when total daily fat consumption climbed to 37% of total caloric intake, it didn't significantly alter total cholesterol or raise LDL (bad) cholesterol.

The research proves coconut oil may also significantly improve blood lipid profile in at-risk patients. The team even suggested that coconut oil be used in increased-risk cardiovascular patients with low HDL cholesterol levels.

## CHAPTER 7

# REVERSE AGING AND LOOK DECADES YOUNGER WITH THE ULTIMATE HEALING FAT OF LIFE

Coconut oil is hands down one of the best healing fats for your brain and your heart. It's the ultimate healing fat of life for a reason. This incredible oil can help you build a better body by strengthening your bones, boosting your antioxidant capacity, transforming your oral health, and even balancing hormones.

In addition to coconut oil's antiviral and antimicrobial properties, it is a stable dry oil that is easily absorbed into your skin.

Coconut oil's remarkable properties help you turn back the clock *internally* and can help you look younger *externally* as well. That's why this is one chapter you'll want to bookmark so you can refer back to it often!

### Renew Your Skin and Treat Skin Problems with the Ideal Moisturizer

If you have dry, rough, scaly, or itchy skin, coconut oil is a centuries old effective moisturizer. It isn't just any old moisturizer...it's also naturally antiseptic!

Research studies from Makati Medical Center, Department of Dermatology in the Philippines, conducted a double-blind controlled clinical trial that patients with xerosis (dry, scaly, rough, and itchy skin). Some participants were given a traditional moisturizer made with mineral oil. Others were given coconut oil. Patients that used coconut oil showed greater improvement in skin texture and overall hydration.

In an 8-week separate study in the Philippines, 117 patients with atopic dermatitis (a chronic skin disease in which the skin's barrier function is compromised and inflamed) were evaluated, as they were treated with either mineral oil or virgin coconut oil. The patients in the virgin coconut oil group showed an improvement in skin quality and inflammation lessened by over 46%!

The virgin coconut oil decreased bacterial *Staph aureus* colonies found on skin by 50%, when applied twice daily in patients affected with chronic skin inflammation.

In addition, massaging coconut oil into your skin can help prevent stretch marks, reduce the appearance, and fade existing stretch marks.

Bonus: Coconut oil is heat stable. That means it can sit in your bathroom for months and won't go rancid. Massage into your skin from head to toe when you get out of the shower and enjoy the skin-enhancing benefits of coconut oil.

## COCONUT OIL HELPS PRETERM BABIES

Preterm babies given a coconut oil massage showed faster weight gain and growth compared to those given a mineral oil massage.

Coconut oil contains the skin nutrient vitamin E, which can help fade age spots and dark underarms. Coconut oil has also been proven to treat:

- Eczema
- Keratosis Polaris
- Psoriasis
- Rosacea
- Hyperpigmentation
- Skin yeast
- Fungal skin infections

## SUMMER SUN SKIN CARE WITH COCONUT OIL

The centuries-old tradition of using coconut oil as sunscreen in tropical nations has legitimate science behind it.

The scare tactics of the sunscreen industry robbed an entire generation of a vital vitamin received from the sun – vitamin D. Over 85% of the U.S. population is vitamin D-deficient which leads to an increased risk of depression, heart disease, diabetes, cancer, and osteoporosis (weak and brittle bones).

Even though too much sun exposure can damage the skin and create premature wrinkles, if you make smart choices about how you soak up sunshine, you can gain the benefits safely.

Stop exposing your skin to toxic sunscreen, which can disrupt your endocrine system. Your skin is your largest organ and you need to protect it. Coconut oil has a natural SPF of between 4-10 and offers excellent hydration to keep your skin from drying out. Adding zinc oxide to coconut oil provides the full spectrum of ultraviolet ray protection without the nasty additives you find on market shelves.

When you've finished getting your sunny dose of vitamin D, apply coconut oil all over your body. Your skin will retain its color and you won't experience the painful blistering and peeling if you spend a bit too much time in the sun. Be smart about the sun, cover up, and enjoy summer!

---

## Transform Your Oral Health with Coconut Oil

There's an old saying that death begins in your gums. Researchers from the University of Otago, Dunedin, New Zealand agreed. They found that your body's own defenses could "overreact" to the threat of gum disease and destroy its own protective cells.

This activity could lead to a buildup of plaque in the arteries that makes them harden, a condition called atherosclerosis, the primary cause of heart attacks. This clearly links the importance of your oral health to your overall wellbeing.

*Every 33 seconds someone in the United States dies from cardiovascular disease. By 2020, heart disease will be the leading cause of death throughout the world.*

Bad dental health has even been proven to lead to pneumonia. Dr. Samit Joshi of the Yale University School of Medicine found that changes in mouth bacteria could increase the risk of developing pneumonia.

Poor oral health has also been associated with:

- Diabetes
- Increased risk of strokes
- Premature births
- Bacterial chest infections
- Metabolic syndrome
- Asthma
- Emphysema
- Osteoporosis
- Chronic bronchitis
- Liver disease
- Arthritis
- HPV infections
- Cancer (cervical, vaginal, penile, throat, tonsils, and base of tongue)

Most dentists recommend regular brushing and flossing to prevent gum disease but you can take oral hygiene one-step further. I want to give you a simple way to transform your oral health. Think of it as a daily oil change for your gums.

In traditional Ayurvedic medicine – one of the world's oldest recorded medical systems – oil pulling was proclaimed to cure as many as 30 systemic diseases.

Oil pulling is a practice that involves swishing or "pulling" oil in the mouth.

A study of 20 subjects by the People's College of Dental Sciences and Research Centre in Bhopal, India reviewed the effects of oil pulling on gingivitis compared to chlorhexidine mouthwash, regularly prescribed by dentists to treat gingivitis.

Oil pulling worked as effectively as the chlorhexidine mouthwash and significantly reduced bad bacteria colony count, plaque, gingivitis, and aerobic microorganisms in just 10 days.

Making coconut oil a far better alternative for oral hygiene than mouthwashes that contain chlorhexidine. This particular chemical has been linked to an increased risk of heart attack according to a recent article in *Free Radical Biology and Medicine*. Along with the bad bacteria, antiseptic mouthwash destroys the beneficial bacteria that are essential to your health.

## Oil Pulling with Coconut Oil

So, are you in love with coconut oil yet?

It is one of the most nutritionally dense superfoods known to man with hundreds of uses and health benefits. One of the reasons it's so special is that it's a natural antimicrobial food.

The healing properties of coconut oil go above and beyond basic nutritional value. Coconut oil can stimulate immune function, increase resistance to infection, and destroy deadly pathogenic microorganisms.

These properties make coconut oil the perfect choice to fight and destroy harmful oral bacteria responsible for tooth decay.

Two components that make coconut oil an antimicrobial food:

Lauric Acid: coconut oil contains the highest concentration of lauric acid of any other substance on earth (about 50%). Your body uses this acid to destroy lipid-coated viruses such as HIV, herpes, influenza, measles, gram-negative bacteria, and protozoa such as giardia lamblia.

Capric Acid: a medium-chain fatty acid found in saturated fats and abundant in coconut oil, capric acid is a strong antiviral and antimicrobial compound.

When ingested, it is converted to monocaprin by your body. It combats viruses, bacteria, and yeast.

Billions of bacteria, viruses, and fungi swarm in your mouth. How lovely is that thought? These bacteria produce toxic by-products, which cause inflammation, weaken tooth enamel, and irritate gums. An overgrowth of dental bacteria can lead to bigger dental problems such as tooth decay and gum disease...and eventually tooth loss.

Start protecting your teeth by oil pulling with coconut oil...

The bacteria in your mouth create a film that adheres to the surface of your teeth. This substance, known as "plaque," is normal but you don't want it get out of hand. Excess plaque eventually hardens and becomes tartar, which can't be brushed away and contributes to gum disease.

You can remove a large amount of bacteria and plaque in your mouth by trying this daily oil pulling technique using coconut oil. Give it a try...it is both simple and effective.

Place a tablespoon of coconut oil in your mouth (it may take a few seconds for it to melt). You may have to start with a smaller amount than a tablespoon and gradually use more.

Swish the oil in your mouth much as you would mouthwash, pushing it around your teeth and against your cheeks.

Do this for at least 3 minutes at first and work your way up. Your goal should be to "swish" the oil for no less than 15 minutes.

Do not swallow the oil! It contains toxins and bacteria gathered from your mouth.

Spit out the oil, rinse with water, and brush your teeth as usual.

Quick tip you might want to use to save time. Try doing oil pulling in the shower on an empty stomach. I recommend spitting out the oil in a trash can since you could clog your pipes if you spit the oil down the drain. Most people prefer doing oil pulling first thing in the morning before they've had anything to eat or drink.

It may seem odd at first but stick with it!

With oil pulling, you'll have fresher breath, a bright white smile, and healthier gums. Teeth are meant to last a lifetime so make sure to take care of them and add this easy oral health technique to your daily routine!

"Inflammation in the mouth is a precursor to inflammation in the body," Dr. Jonathan Levine, D.D.S.

## Create the Mother of All Anti-Aging Antioxidants with Coconut Oil

The antioxidant I'm going to talk about now is the most important molecule you will ever need. It's the key to preventing aging, dementia, heart disease, cancer, kidney disease, autoimmune diseases, diabetes, and every conceivable health condition known to man.

It's been called "the mother of all antioxidants" for many reasons. This incredible compound is called **glutathione**.

Glutathione acts as a detoxification agent for your body and as an immune system booster. Without it, you would suffer from rapid cell disintegration from free radicals and infections.

As critical as it is to your very life, this powerful amino acid doesn't get much love.

The good news is your body produces glutathione (pronounced "gloot-a-thigh-own"). When your body creates enough of it, toxins don't stand a chance. Taking a glutathione supplement usually doesn't work because it doesn't make it past the digestive fluids in your stomach to the liver where you need it most.

Foods rich in sulfur can boost your glutathione levels.

- Kale
- Onions
- Garlic
- Cauliflower
- Broccoli
- Asparagus
- Avocados
- Grass-fed beef
- Grass-fed butter

Another antioxidant that boosts your body's defenses against disease is **superoxide dismutase**. What's so special about superoxide dismutase (SOD)? SOD is second only to glutathione in its ability to reduce oxidative stress. This protective protein plays a crucial role in reducing internal inflammation, atherosclerosis (hardening of the arteries), stroke, and chronic pain caused by conditions such as arthritis.

Both SOD and glutathione can be a challenge taking via supplementation, as the digestive process easily deactivates the enzyme and amino acid.

A study by the Department of Biochemistry, University of Kerala, India in September 2013 confirmed that wet-milled virgin coconut oil increased the antioxidant formation of glutathione, glutathione peroxidase, and superoxide dismutase (SOD).

Wet-milled virgin coconut oil is a traditional method of producing coconut oil. The coconut is crushed, made into a slurry, and squeezed through a cheesecloth to make coconut milk.

The milk is refrigerated for 48 hours, and then subjected to mild heat. Virgin coconut oil is filtered through a cheesecloth using this low-tech method.

Since coconut oil is a heat stable oil, the low-level heat used produces a higher polyphenol antioxidant level in this form of the oil than in the unheated versions. This does not mean that unheated virgin coconut oil is unhealthy. The difference is only in the higher antioxidant level. It does not change the fatty acid structure at all.

Glutathione levels were significantly increased in just 6 weeks in the liver, heart, and kidneys – preventing and reducing oxidative stress to primary organs simply by adding virgin coconut oil to the diet.

## Stay Young Inside: Create Stronger Bones Today

Lipid peroxidation is a huge factor in oxidative stress. Free radicals form from polyunsaturated oils that aren't shelf stable. The major ones used in U.S. food production are corn and soybean oil.

When you combine the oxidative stress increase with the fact that these two crops are also genetically modified more than 90% of the time and you have a recipe for several chronic conditions generated from reactive oxygen species including osteoporosis, osteoarthritis, and rheumatoid arthritis.

Virgin coconut oil has the highest polyphenol content hands down. This helps the phenolic acids scavenge and destroy free radicals that create oxidative stress and lipid peroxidation. Malondialdehyde (MDA) is the marker for oxidative stress generated from reactive oxygen species (ROS) and these degenerative conditions.

Consumption of virgin coconut oil significantly reduced MDA level, increased SOD level, and prevented lipid peroxidation within the bone, which may prevent osteoporotic bone damage.

# CHAPTER 8
# HEALING FATS... THE ULTIMATE HORMONE BALANCER

Your endocrine system is a group of little-known glands that you might not think about often. It's a special group of organs and cells that make the hormones that your body needs.

The endocrine system regulates:

- Metabolism
- Sexual function
- Reproduction
- Mood
- Growth and development

In addition to the hormones found in both genders, men produce specific hormones in their testes and women produce them in their ovaries and uterus.

Hormones are created by using good fats and cholesterol. Therefore, when these two important dietary factors are lacking then hormone problems can rage out of control.

If you've been eating a diet filled with polyunsaturated toxic oils and chemicals, then your body doesn't have the proper building blocks it needs to make these hormones. Worse, your body could be using the *wrong* building blocks and no one wants mutant hormones running around.

Oxidized fats found in vegetable oils contain polyunsaturated fats. The human body is about 97% saturated fat and monounsaturated fat and only 3% polyunsaturated fat.

Yet with vegetable oils replacing saturated fats naturally found in virgin coconut oil, red palm oil, lard, tallow, suet, and grass-fed butter, we have create an environment that causes inflammation and mutation in cells.

These mutations damage reproductive tissue, creating problems such as endometriosis (the painful buildup of tissue on the walls of your uterus) and polycystic ovary syndrome (PCOS) (small cysts grow on the ovaries – a condition that is the leading cause of infertility in women). They also create clogged arteries and skin cancer.

Virgin coconut oil is astounding for hormonal health and balance. It provides the necessary building blocks in the form of fatty acids and cholesterol. Particularly lauric acid, which is extremely beneficial for hormone production.

Most of the saturated fat in our diets comes in one of four varieties: lauric acid, myristic, acid, stearic acid, and palmitic acid. Coconut oil contains all of these and is especially abundant in lauric, capric, and myristic acids.

- Lauric acid: Antibacterial, natural antibiotic, and immune system booster
- Capric acid: Prevents viral infections
- Myristic acid: Protects gums and helps liver synthesize cholesterol
- Stearic acid: Skin protectant, antioxidant and antibacterial properties
- Palmitic acid: Cardiovascular protection

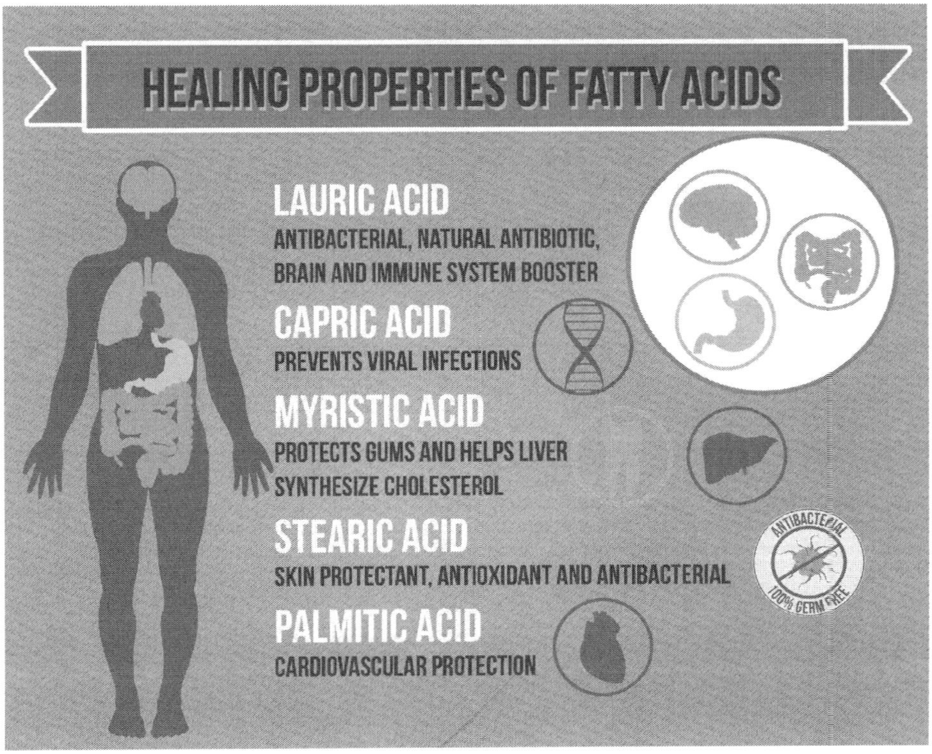


As for the men...coconut oil was found to have two beneficial effects on male prostate health.

Enlarged prostate or benign prostatic hyperplasia (BPH) affects nearly 50% of men over the age of 60 and nearly 90% of all men report symptoms by age 85. Coconut oil has been found to reduce benign prostate growth by 28%.

Coconut oil is also fantastic for boosting testosterone by reducing the level of oxidative stress in the testes. This healing fat also showed the highest levels of antioxidants in the testicles when compared to soybean oil, olive oil, and grapeseed oil.

By adding at least two tablespoons of coconut oil to your diet every day, you provide your body a safe and natural way to balance your hormones, maintain your bone strength, and keep your skin looking young and fresh.

## Free Testosterone Crucial to Your Health

Have you heard of free testosterone? No, it isn't being given away out of the back of a van.

Free testosterone is the amount of unattached testosterone found in your bloodstream. Most of the testosterone in your blood attaches to certain proteins. The unattached or "free" testosterone flows in your blood.

Since both men and women produce this vital sex hormone and it's responsible for sexual traits, it's important to know how free testosterone can affect your hormones and your health.

A study published in the International Journal of Clinical Practice found that more than 12 million men suffer from lower testosterone and hormone issues but have no idea that the problem exists. As men age their levels of testosterone can fall. By age 60, many men may have less than half the level of testosterone than they did when they were teenagers.

In men, low levels of free testosterone can create these health risks:

- Metabolic syndrome
- Type 2 diabetes
- Heart disease
- Cancer
- Anemia
- Depression
- Fatigue
- Loss of muscle mass
- Poor concentration
- Erectile dysfunction
- Infertility
- Earlier death
- Hypothyroidism

Whether you are man or a woman, you want the optimal level of free testosterone flowing through your blood.

Around 4% to 7% of women produce too much testosterone in their ovaries. Women that have elevated levels of testosterone and androgen hormones often suffer from polycystic ovary syndrome PCOS and have high levels of insulin and insulin resistance.

In women, elevated levels of free testosterone can create these health risks:

- Cystic acne

- Excess hair growth
- Polycystic ovary syndrome (PCOS)
- Infertility
- Lack of menstruation

To balance female hormone levels eliminate processed sugar, junk food, soy products, and starchy carbohydrates. By adding in the healing fats of life to your daily diet, you will find that it can help you to reduce and even eliminate these health risks.

**The Healing Fats of Life Can Help Balance Hormones and Optimize Testosterone Levels**

Researchers at the Center for Sports Medicine at Pennsylvania State University studied the influence of diets on testosterone levels in twelve men. Each subject kept a food journal for seventeen days.

It was found that there was a negative connection to high protein intake and free testosterone levels while there was a positive connection between fat intakes and testosterone levels.

In another study from the University of Cambridge School of Medicine (Cambridge, United Kingdom) tracked more than 11,600 British men for up to 10 years. The researchers found that men in the upper 25% of natural testosterone levels have a 41% lower risk of dying from heart attack, stroke and other cardiovascular conditions, cancers and all other causes (compared to men with the lowest levels of testosterone).

The research team said, "Low testosterone seems to predict increased risk of total mortality in cardiovascular disease and cancer."

Since fat and cholesterol are the precursors for creating testosterone, if you don't eat enough dietary fats, you won't be able to produce adequate levels of any sex hormones.

Now that you are getting to know, the different types of healing fats that your body needs - the quality of the fats you consume matters most.

The best sources of saturated and monounsaturated healing fats for optimal testosterone levels are organic coconut oil, organic grass fed butter, ghee, tallow, lard, free-range eggs, cacao butter, avocados, and grass fed beef.

Avoid chemically created fats found in vegetable oils, margarine, peanut oil, canola oil, corn oil, cottonseed oil, safflower oil, sunflower oil, or soybean oil, that are high in omega-6 polyunsaturated fats. These deadly fats create inflammation, lower testosterone levels and can create problems like endometriosis and PCOS in women.

The exception to this rule are polyunsaturated fatty acids with high omega-3 content, such as – wild salmon, wild fish, cod liver oil, fermented cod liver oil, krill oil, olive oil, brazil nuts, and walnuts.

In addition to boosting testosterone and balancing hormones naturally with healing fats, adding the following health practices can help both men and women:

- Lift heavy weights (dumbbells, kettle bells, barbells) and do squats. Aim for shorter high intensity workouts.
- Eat foods rich in vitamin D and zinc – oysters, shellfish, antibiotic / hormone free eggs and meats.
- Get adequate sleep, more than six hours each night.
- Don't smoke.
- Reduce your sugar intake.
- Reduce alcohol consumption – alcohol raises cortisol levels and inhibits growth hormones, which lowers testosterone levels. (Beer is the worst offender, since hops used are full of estrogen.)
- Don't eat too much protein. If you consume excessive protein then your body converts the leftover protein into glucose and stores it as body fat if not used.
- Avoid heating food in plastic containers. Most plastics contain phthalates (a type of xenoestrogen) and bisphenol-A (BPA), which can be transferred to your food when plastic is heated. Use glass containers when possible. Even if the plastic containers you use are BPA-free, most of the time BPA has been replaced with a similar plastic that has the same endocrine system - disrupting effect.

# CHAPTER 9

# IT'S TRUE... FAT DOESN'T MAKE YOU FAT

Fat got a bad rap. It doesn't contribute to heart disease, it doesn't raise cholesterol, and it doesn't harm your body. You now know the exact opposite is the case – your body *needs* and *craves* fat.

I'll show you the real culprit behind what's really making you fat. I've touched on it earlier chapters, but if you are struggling with your weight, whether you need to lose 10 pounds or 100 pounds, these studies and the proof offered will change how you approach losing weight forever.

The science isn't new...when Dr. Robert Atkin's came out with his revolutionary diet of high fat low carbohydrates in 1972, the population felt as if they'd received Willie Wonka's golden ticket to diet on nothing but steak.

A year later, a disturbed American Congress summoned him to a hearing about fad diets. He was labeled as a quack! How dare he tell Americans the opposite of what the establishment had been telling them for decades? The "party line" was that the only way to lose weight was by avoiding fat and eating a lot of grains.

Atkin's had a flair for the dramatic. He decided that he was going to be the best enemy the establishment had. Since the evidence-based medicine at the time was in opposition to Atkin's findings, he focused on experiential medicine. He tried different things with his patients and continued to do what worked for them.

Your diet is a lifestyle issue and it is as much a part of your social life as it is a medical issue. Eating rich high-fat foods with delicious vegetables, or consuming coconut oil straight off the spoon the way I do for breakfast...it seems plain *wrong* to most folks.

On the other hand, if you're suffering with counting calories – living off dry toast and a small bowl of whole-wheat pasta – does that seem okay? Where's the joy living in such a way? Where's the science behind those claims?

The culprit making our collective waistline expand to epidemic proportions isn't fat...it is carbohydrates.

## It's Not Fat's Fault: How Carbohydrates Make You Sick and Fat

Simple processed carbohydrates are responsible for obesity in America. The trouble begins in your mind before you take the first bite.

When you *think* about a meal containing carbohydrates, your body begins to secrete insulin. The signal goes out for fatty acids to be stored and conserve energy. You get hungry, you eat that bowl of pasta or that low-fat muffin, and you secrete more insulin. he digested carbohydrates enter your bloodstream as glucose and your blood sugar levels rise, causing your body to secrete insulin *again* to control it.

Foods made from refined flour – such as pasta, cereals, and breads that we consume at insane levels – are the worst offenders. Equally dangerous to your waistline are beer, fruit juice, soda, corn, potatoes, and rice. These easily digestible carbohydrates are the most fattening.

Now your pancreas is in high gear and sends out a flood of insulin to deal with all the excess glucose pumping through your bloodstream.

Maybe you start to feel a little nervous, spastic, or even "high" depending on how many carbs you ate – especially if it was something like birthday cake.

All that glucose needs somewhere to go. If your glycogen stores have room then some of the sugar goes into your muscles. If you don't have the space (most of us don't due to this process repeating multiple times a day), the excess marches right into several other tissues, where it's **stored as fat**.

Your body doesn't realize that you ate cookies, a sugary coffee drink, a bowl of pasta, or a slice of pizza. No, it feels (and responds) as if your entire system is under attack. The sense of "emergency" creates a rush of adrenaline and a spike of cortisol. You get some "feel good" hormones as well to level things out.

An hour or two later, the rush is gone and you start to feel sluggish and tired. That's the arrival of the sugar crash.

Congratulations! You've unintentionally wreaked havoc on your entire immune system. If you're like the majority of the Western world, this series of events will happen more than once every single day because our diet guarantees it.

*More cookies anyone?*

Your immune system phagocyte cells protect the body by eating bacteria, dying cells, foreign bodies, and protozoa. Research proves that after the intake of simple sugars glucose, fructose, sucrose, orange juice, and even honey...phagocyte function is impaired for at least five hours.

That is five hours that your immune system is "offline" and unresponsive to real threats. Much the way watching a funny video can crash your computer and make it impossible for you to finish that urgent report due by noon.

Researchers from Stanford University put one group of people on a low-carb diet high in fat and protein and another group on a low-fat diet high in carbohydrates. The group on the low-carb diet lost an average of 9.9 pounds where the group on low-fat diet lost around 5.5 pounds.

*What makes us fat?* Carbohydrates. The process even has a name: **de novo lipogenesis** (DNL) – the act of your body turning carbohydrates into fat.

Blood sugar rises and triggers the manufacture of fat through de novo lipogenesis and secondarily by triggering insulin that reduces fat breakdown. This creates fat accumulation because your body *makes* more fat while using less fat.

Fat is stored in cells in the form of triglycerides. These triglycerides are formed by three fatty acids bound to one molecule of glycerol. Fatty acids are able to flow through your body freely. Anything that promotes the flow of fatty acids

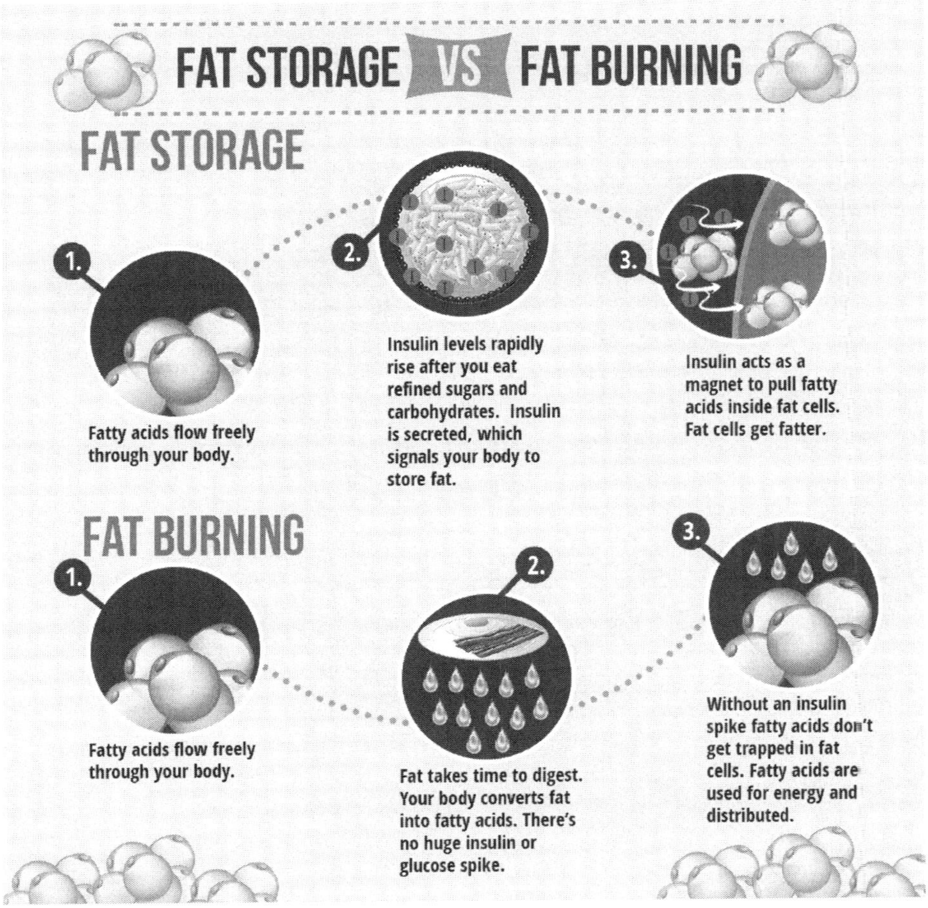

into your cells gets stored as fat. Anything that helps breakdown triglycerides makes you leaner and helps you lose weight.

Insulin is the primary watchdog of fat metabolism and LPL (lipoprotein lipase – a fat regulator) sits on the membrane of cells and acts as a magnet to pull fat inside. The more insulin we secrete, the more active LPL is on our fat cells.

When insulin levels rise after we eat refined sugars and carbohydrates, we store fat. Insulin inhibits the breakdown of fat (adipose) tissue. Then insulin levels drop and we use that fat for fuel.

Carbohydrates spike insulin levels and rising insulin creates fat accumulation. The types of carbohydrates we consume are what determine how much fat we accumulate.

## The Metabolic Benefits of Eating Healing Fats

- Stimulates healthy weight loss
- Leads to fat loss because fat is used as fuel instead of stored in fat cells
- Improves blood triglycerides – a key bio-marker for cardiovascular disease
- Improves HDL (good) cholesterol levels – another key bio-marker for cardiovascular disease
- Changes the size of LDL (bad) cholesterol into larger particles - easier for the body to process and flush
- Ketone production and utilization increases in the body
- Gluconeogenesis (making of new glucose) decreases
- Helps reverse non-alcoholic fatty liver disease (NAFLD) which is an increasing problem since your liver is the processing center for the body and extremely vulnerable to metabolic syndrome (high blood sugar, high blood fats, inflammation, and insulin resistance)
- Manages adrenal response and the production of cortisol (which increases appetite, sugar cravings, and weight gain) – preventing your cells from being flooded with glucose

Dr. Eric Westman, director of the Duke University Obesity Clinic, is pleased that mainstream media is finally debunking the myth that eating fat makes you fat and sick. To the contrary, he stated, "Eating fat makes you skinny and healthy."

Author of "*A New Atkins for a New You*," Dr. Westman continues, "I tell my patients not to fear the fat. Eat lots of fat. Fat makes you feel full. There's no problem with fat. In fact, saturated fat, the fat that we've been taught not to eat, raises your good cholesterol best of all the foods you can eat."

When evaluating what diet right for you, look far beyond your need to lose weight. Think about how it affects your overall health and total body wellness.

Does it increase your vitality? Does it change dangerous metabolic markers? Does it (most importantly) help reverse your risk of chronic disease?

Your body *loves* healing fats. By adding them to your diet, your waistline will thank you, your liver will breathe a sigh of relief, and you'll stay vibrant and healthy for years to come!

# CHAPTER 10

# THE SCIENCE OF CENTURIES-OLD HEALING FATS

In the early 1900s, only 1-in-150 people were considered obese. By 1971, the obesity rate increased to 14% (14-in-100 people). Right now, a little more than 40 years later, the national obesity rate has hit a whopping 34% (34-in-100 people)!

The obesity rate is projected to hit 42% by 2050...and none of these figures include the statistics for the portion of the population that is merely considered "overweight."

What has changed?

As a society, we are no longer eating real whole foods. Instead, we eat manufactured foodstuffs laced with sugar, refined flours, and chemical based salts.

Let's make a pact to get back to eating real foods and using the centuries-old healing fats our grandparent's used. They ate lard and didn't have the epidemics of obesity, heart disease, Alzheimer's, and cancer that plague us today. These diseases were very rare before the 1900s.

*What's that you say?* They lived shorter lives? Not really. In the 1900's infant mortality rate was at an all-time high due to unsanitary medical conditions.

If you look at total human lifespan versus life expectancy, you'll see that it's remained constant for thousands of years. When Socrates died at the age of 70 in 399 B.C., it wasn't due to old age...he was executed. It seems strange that ancient Greeks lived into their 70s and beyond but 2000 years later, we aren't living that much longer.

In fact, the Victorians of England were better nourished than we are today. They ate eight to ten portions of vegetables daily and consumed large quantities of meat and game. Sugar was rarely consumed. The average life expectancy was 75 for men and 73 for women.

Treat these healing fats with love and use them in moderation and you'll see the benefits of adding them into your daily life.

## The Creamy Goodness of Lard

Let's talk about lard or rendered pork fat. My Grandma loves lard. She would render her own and to her, it was beautiful creamy fatty goodness.

It's not difficult to render your own lard but if you don't have the time, then pastured lard is nutrient-dense, a great source of vitamin D, and 48% mono-unsaturated fat. It contains the same fatty acid found in olive oil. It's odd that lard is beaten up while olive oil is praised.

Back in the early 1900s, Proctor & Gamble made a mint in cotton production. The cottonseed was a pesky by-product of cotton and they decided to see if there was any way that they could make a profit from it.

After a lot of processing and heat extraction – they extracted oil that costs almost nothing to produce. Cottonseed oil was extremely unstable regarding shelf life so they hydrogenated it…and Crisco™ was born. When it cooled, it looked exactly like lard.

Proctor & Gamble's decision to market this by-product of cotton production turned the tide against lard that had been used for thousands of years and created a lot sickness and disease in the process. Lard was suddenly too smelly, too messy and P&G created cookbooks that substituted their Crisco™ for lard and butter.

Cotton is not considered a food crop by the United States Food and Drug Administration (FDA) and it does not fall under pesticide usage regulations. In fact, more pesticides are sprayed on cotton than any other crop! Before processing, cottonseed is toxic for human and animal consumption.

An issue from the *Popular Science* of the era says it plainly, "What was garbage in 1860 was fertilizer in 1870, cattle feed in 1880, and table food and many things else in 1890."

Cottonseed oil is over 50% omega-6 fatty acids and kicks off your inflammatory response. You could make coconut oil at home, you could make lard, you can even make olive oil, but there's no way you can create cottonseed oil in your kitchen.

Why would you want to eat something that can only be created in a lab?

Lard is not only a healthier option, it was probably your grandparent's favorite healing fat (and they didn't even know it).

One tablespoon of lard contains 1000 IU of vitamin D. Vitamin D can usually only be metabolized through sun exposure. After just 15 minutes of sun exposure to bare skin, you'll receive around 10,000 IUs of vitamin D (the minutes you need depend on your skin type, time of year, and air quality of where you live).

Sun exposure is far more difficult if you live in a cold climate, during the winter months in much of the world, or if you have a special sensitivity to UV rays.

Lard is an excellent alternate source of vitamin D that is available year-round. Vitamin D can be found in trace amounts in fatty fish but the only plant sources of vitamin D are some mushrooms that provide 21 IUs. You'd have to eat around 50 mushrooms to match the benefit of one tablespoon of lard.

Vitamin D is a powerful immune booster that can help prevent cold and flu. It helps with calcium absorption that improves bone and oral health. Then there is vitamin D's crucial role in hormone production and regulation. Not to mention the helping hand it lends to heavy metal detoxification.

Vitamin D deficiency has been linked to adrenal problems with fibromyalgia, thyroid issues through hypothyroidism, and sex hormone problems through infertility.

The main fat content of lard is oleic acid, a fatty acid that decreases the risk of depression. A Thailand Study found that oleic acid (an omega-9 fatty acid) also reduced the risk of breast cancer by blocking the action of a cancer causing oncogene. It lowers your risk of heart disease, reduces LDL (bad) cholesterol levels, and leaves HDL (good) cholesterol alone.

If you purchase lard, be sure it isn't hydrogenated or produced from pigs in concentrated animal feeding operations (CAFO).

It's relatively easy to make yourself and you'll have an easier time finding a farmer, butcher, or meat shop that raises pastured or foraged pigs. A pig raised outside, soaking up the sun, is one reason why lard is so high in vitamin D.

Lard is natural and sustainable. It makes everything taste delicious, even simple foods such as cauliflower hash browns and eggs are elevated to a new level when you cook with lard.

**How to Render Lard on Your Stove Top**

YIELD: 1/2 - gallon

Ensure you have a high quality, heavy-bottomed stockpot. Two and one-half pounds of fresh leaf lard or hog fat will produce approximately one-half gallon of creamy, nutrient-dense fat.

Ingredients

- 2 ½ pounds pastured leaf lard or hog fat
- ½ cup filtered water

Instructions

With a sharp knife, trim any blood spots or remaining meat from the lard.

Chop the fat into ½-inch cubes.

Add the chopped fat and the filtered water to a heavy-bottomed stockpot and simmer over medium-low heat, stirring occasionally.

After 45-60 minutes, the water will evaporate and the fat will begin to melt. The cracklings – little bits of browned fat – will begin to float to the surface. Continue to stir the melted fat periodically, taking care not to let it splatter.

When the cracklings sink to the bottom of the stockpot, remove your pot from the heat.

Line a fine mesh sieve with a 100% cotton cheesecloth and strain the melted fat, reserving the cracklings for another use (they're quite nice salted and eaten as a snack or served in place of breadcrumbs in a gratin).

Pour the melted fat into mason jars and allow to cool. The melted fat will be golden-brown in color, but, when cooled, will appear a creamy white.

Use your freshly rendered lard in pastries, as a fat for braising vegetables and seasoning meats.

Adapted from Nourished Kitchen

## An Ayurvedic Healing Fat: Ghee

In ancient Ayurveda, the milk of cows is considered to possess the spirit of all plants and ghee is the essence of milk.

Ghee is derived from the Sanskrit word meaning "sprinkled" and literally means that milk fat is rendered from butter to separate the milk solids and water.

This healing fat is essentially clarified butter made by heating butter and skimming the fat off the top. When the simple process is finished, you'll have a golden liquid. Once it cools, it turns into a creamy solid.

The beauty of ghee is that if you're lactose intolerant or have dairy allergies you'll get the benefits of butterfat without lactose and casein. It tastes fabulous and is a stable fat with a very high smoke point of 450°F/230°C.

Ghee doesn't spoil easily. There are records of some ghee mixtures lasting as long as 100 years.

Ghee is so highly regarded in India that it is even said, "*Eating Ghee is like offering the finest fuels into the fires of digestion.* In earliest Ayurvedic healing records, ghee was used to:

- Build the aura
- Make organs soft
- Build the internal "juices" of the body, that aging destroys
- Increase digestion
- Refine the intellect
- Improve memory
- Carry away toxins
- Create longevity

In ancient times, ghee was rubbed on wounds, used for peptic ulcers, to heal bedsores, applied to broken bones and bruises, used on skin rashes, and even applied to burns.

Science now proves that ghee is a superfood. You can use ghee to sauté or stir-fry.

Ghee is rich in vitamin K2 (the essential heart nutrient) and in conjugated linoleic acid (CLA) (an antiviral and antioxidant compound). CLA has been shown to help fight cancer and aid in weight loss.

If you have a troublesome gut, ghee converts fiber into butyric acid, which is beneficial for intestinal bacteria. Various lab studies show that ghee reduces serum and intestine cholesterol. It helps brain and nerve function.

## How to Make Your Own Ghee

Ingredients

- 1 lbs. grass fed butter
- Skillet with high sides
- Fine mesh skimmer and strainer or cheesecloth
- Glass jar, container, or Mason jar for storage

Instructions

Heat a wide-bottomed skillet with high sides (for splashing/bubbling) over medium-low heat. Once hot, add butter.

Use a wooden spoon or spatula to stir the butter and speed along the melting process.

Once butter is completely melted and begins to bubble, very slightly lower the heat. You want a steady bubble but not so much that butter is jumping out of the pan or spraying on the stovetop.

Cook 25-30 minutes or until the milk protein has completely separated and there is a layer on the top and bits on the bottom of the pan.

Begin carefully skimming the top layer off until the ghee looks clean (except for bits on the very bottom) and discard.

Slightly raise the heat back to medium low and continue cooking another 5-10 minutes until most of the bubbling stops and the milk protein bits on the bottom of the pan begin to brown. Do not let them burn!

Immediately remove the ghee from the stovetop and set somewhere to cool.

Once cool, strain through a fine mesh strainer or cheesecloth. Discard the toasted bits from the bottom of the pan.

Store ghee at room temperature in a glass container or Mason jar and use as needed.

Recipe Adapted from Everyday Maven

## How Conjugated Linoleic Acid (CLA) Protects Your Health

Conjugated linoleic acid is related to the omega-6 fatty acids that help the body increase metabolic rates, boost immunity, and keep cholesterol levels regulated.

In the late 1980s, Professor Michael Pariza of the University of Wisconsin discovered an isolated agent in fried hamburger that reduced cancer in mice. A few years later, his team identified the compound as CLA.

One consistent finding in the avalanche of studies on CLA that followed was that it helped people lose body fat. A Norwegian study published in 2000 found that CLA reduced body fat and preserved muscle in overweight or obese people. The CLA group – despite not changing their diet – lost six more pounds of body fat than those in the placebo group.

CLA reduces body fat by increasing basal metabolic rates. It also keeps fat cells from expanding, which alters the fat-to-muscle ratio.

Dr. Delbert Dorscheid, a cancer and asthma researcher, discovered that:

- Women with increased levels of CLA have lower breast cancer rates
- Same findings reported for colon and prostate cancer
- Overall decrease in cardiovascular disease
- Reversed type 2 diabetes

According to Dr. Joseph Mercola, some of the best possible sources of CLA are grass-fed beef and raw dairy products that come from grass-fed cattle.

Studies from the U.S. Dairy Forage Research Center in Madison, Wisconsin found that cows grazing pasture and receiving no supplemental feed had 500% more conjugated linoleic acid in their milk fat than cows fed typical dairy diets of hay, fishmeal, grain, and alfalfa silage. Keeping cattle on a natural diet such as grass, levels of CLA are 3-5 times more than those fed on grain based diet. Bottom line, grass-fed is better than grain-fed beef for human health.

Always make sure your butter is from pastured or grass fed cows and that it is free of hormones and antibiotics.

On the other hand, if you want to make your own ghee, purchase the best grass-fed butter you can find. Preferably local, if you can find it at a farmer's market or natural food store.

## Healing Fat: Tallow

If you haven't heard of tallow, it's a rendered healing fat made from beef or suet. It's technically the same as lard but it comes from a cow instead of a pig.

Did you know...McDonald's French fries used to be fried in beef tallow until 1990, when they switched to partially hydrogenated vegetable oil?

Even Julia Child complained of the change to vegetable oil in 1990. She said, "The nutritionists got at them, which turned out to be erroneous and said beef tallow and lard were bad. So they changed it to some kind of nutritionist oil and they just got kind of limp and I've never eaten them ever since."

Dr. Weston A. Price – famed researcher, dentist, and nutritionist – investigated traditional diets versus civilized diets. His findings revealed that once native peoples left their traditional ways of eating and switched to diets high in refined sugars, starches, and seed oils, they succumbed to heart disease, diabetes, and other chronic diseases.

Tallow is made from the fat of the kidney and loin area of the cow. It is over 56% saturated fat and has a high smoke point as well. For high-heat cooking this is one of the best fats to use because it remains stable and doesn't generate free radicals when heated.

Grass-fed beef tallow gives you the benefits of CLA and tallow is a superb source of:

- Niacin
- Vitamins B6, B12, K2
- Selenium
- Iron
- Phosphorous
- Potassium
- Riboflavin

### The Cancer Protective Effects of Beef Tallow

Beef tallow is protective against metastatic breast tumors. Research conducted at The Department of Cell Biology and Human Anatomy, University of California, School of Medicine, Davis, California, showed that "Beef Tallow Increases the Potency of Conjugated Linoleic Acid in the Reduction of Mouse Mammary Tumor Metastasis."

The title says it all. This study showed that mice fed CLA (conjugated linoleic acid) with beef tallow, had fewer metastatic breast tumors than another group that was fed vegetable fat blend. The authors concluded that the fatty acids in beef tallow actually enhanced the (known) anti-tumor actions of CLA.

The authors stated, "Fatty acids normally found in beef tallow, such as oleic, stearic, and palmitic acids, either did not change or enhanced the cytolytic effects of CLA isomers on mouse mammary tumor cells in culture. These data provide evidence that dietary BT, itself with negligible levels of CLA, may increase the efficacy of dietary CLA in reducing mammary tumorigenesis."

**How to Render Beef Tallow**

Ingredients

- 5 pounds of beef fat (suet) and trimmings
- Water (see below for amount)

Instructions

Take a deep heavy-bottomed pot and fill with approximately 2" of water.

Place the entire 5 pounds of fat into the pot and let it melt down on high heat. Turn the heat down to med/high when the melted fat starts to bubble and the impurities rise to the top.

Turn down the heat the lowest temperature you can while keeping the melted fat at a low simmer.

After a few hours, the water will evaporate leaving you with beautiful golden oil. With clear liquid at the bottom and crispy bits floating on top.

Take a stainless steel bowl, set a stainless steel colander on it, line with cheesecloth, and pour the hot oil through (be very careful not to burn yourself). The cloth will catch the fine particles of meat.

Pour into glass jars, containers, or mason jars or line a baking pan with parchment paper and pour liquid fat into the pans.

Allow it to harden completely.

Once the tallow hardens, you can chop it into bars if you used pans. Try frying sweet potatoes, zucchini, or eggplant in it!

## Healing Fats: Poultry and Game

### Chicken Fat (Schmaltz)

Turns out Bubbie's chicken fat (or schmaltz) was good for you after all. Chicken fat was the go-to ingredient for Ashkenazi Jews who had little or no access to olive oil that Jews in the Middle East were accustomed to using in their cooking.

Since cooking meat with butter or lard is considered non-kosher, schmaltz was valued as a reliable stable cooking fat for most German, Austrian, and Polish Jews.

Chicken fat is about 31% saturated, 49% monounsaturated (includes moderate amounts of antimicrobial palmitoleic acid), and 20% polyunsaturated.

### Duck and Goose Fat

The French Paradox is alive and well.

In the United States, 315 of every 100,000 middle-aged men die of heart attacks each year. In France, the rate is 145 per 100,000. In the Gascony region, where goose and duck fat reign supreme, the rate is only 80 per 100,000.

They eat more fat but have less heart disease...coincidence? *I think not.* Dr. Serge Renaud, Director Research at the National Institute of Health and Medical Research, a Government center in Lyons, based these findings off his 10-year study in 1991.

It turns out goose and duck fat are closer in chemical composition to olive oil than to butter or lard. Using fat was one of the first ways to preserve food. It's now a delicacy that we refer to as "confit" that can be sealed and stored for months.

"If we can label *foie gras* health food, ah, the world is then ours," said Jean Michel Justumus, director of the Regional Center for Agricultural and Technological Innovation in Auch, the capital of Gers. The center studies the technology of *foie gras* growing and processing.

Both duck and goose fat are semisolid at room temperature, containing about 35% saturated fat, 52% monounsaturated fat (including small amounts of antimicrobial palmitoleic acid), and about 13% polyunsaturated fat. The proportion of omega-6 to omega-3 fatty acids depends on what the birds have eaten. Duck and goose fat are quite stable.

It turns out *foie gras* isn't to be feared, but rather loved by your heart.

## Lamb Fat

Nearly 2,000 years ago, the Greeks and Romans brought sheep to England and later sheep journeyed to North America with the Spanish in 1519. From Asia to New Zealand, lamb is a revered food.

Nearly half of the fat in lamb is unsaturated. Only 36% of the fat in lamb is saturated.

Lamb contains the brain nutrient arachidonic acid and is one of the richest sources of CLA.

Lamb fat is also a great source of B vitamins, iron, and zinc essential for growth, healing, and a healthy immune system. Lamb is nature's best source for an amino acid called carnitine, which is needed to generate energy from fatty acids.

It has a stronger (or gamier) flavor than other healing fats so start with a little and see if you like the flavor profile. Lamb fat can be rendered in the same way you would beef fat to get lamb tallow.

The health benefits of healing fats like lard and tallow are:

- Enhance the immune system
- Build and strengthen bones and teeth (preventing cavities and osteoporosis)
- Provide energy and structural integrity to the cells
- Protect the liver
- Enhance the body's use of essential fatty acids
- Do not become rancid easily
- Do not call upon the body's reserves of antioxidants
- Do not initiate cancer
- Do not irritate the artery walls

**Fats are the most important aspect of your diet.**

Using these healing fats will help you experience the next level of health and vitality. They provide critical the cholesterol your body requires to repair cell damage. Cholesterol is produced in the liver and used throughout your body – especially your brain, which is 25% cholesterol.

A diet high in polyunsaturated fats causes an imbalance at the cellular level, making your building blocks "flabby" rather than strong and flexible.

Cholesterol is essential to your tissues, your hormones, and vitamin absorption. There is no end to the role it plays inside your body. Depriving yourself of this primary element will lead to heart disease, cancer, neurodegenerative diseases like Alzheimer's, thyroid conditions, and even changes to your mental state.

Fat is not the enemy – you simply require the right kinds of fat in your diet.

Over 100 years ago, these healing fats were used in everyday cooking and heart disease was non-existent. Now heart disease is the number one silent killer in the United States.

The first recorded heart attack was in 1921, just 10 short years after Crisco was introduced to the American public.

You've got the facts...you know that's no coincidence.

Now that you know the power of healing fats, let's keep the tide turning, and start a fat revolution for better health.

## Reference Chart: Smoke Points of Fats

| TYPE OF FAT | SMOKE POINT | REFINED |
|---|---|---|
| Clarified Butter | 450°F/230°C | No |
| Beef Tallow | 400°F/250°C | No |
| Lard | 370°F/185°C | No |
| Avocado Oil (Virgin) | 375-400°F/190-205°C | No |
| Chicken Fat (Schmaltz) | 375°F/190°C | No |
| Duck Fat | 375°F/190°C | No |
| Butter | 350°F/175°C | No |
| Coconut Oil | 350°F/175°C | No |
| Extra-Virgin Olive Oil | 325-375°F/165-190°C | No |

# REFERENCES


Agero, A., & Verallo-Rowell, V. (2004). A Randomized Double-Blind Controlled Trial Comparing Extra Virgin Coconut Oil With Mineral Oil As A Moisturizer For Mild To Moderate Xerosis. *Dermatitis (formerly American Journal of Contact Dermatitis),* 109-109.

Albert Sanchez, J. L. Reeser, H. S. Lau, P. Y. Yahiku, R. E. Willard,P. J. McMillan, S. Y. Cho, A. R. Magie, and U. D. Register. Role of sugars in human neutrophilic phagocytosis. (1973, November). *The American Journal of Clinical Nutrition.*

A.R. Oyi, J.A. Onaolapo and R.C. Obi. (2010) Formulation and Antimicrobial Studies of Coconut (Cocos nucifera Linne) Oil. *Research Journal of Applied Sciences, Engineering and Technology*. 2(2): 133-137.

Arruzazabala, M., Molina, V., Más, R., Carbajal, D., Marrero, D., González, V., & Rodríguez, E. (2007). Effects of coconut oil on testosterone-induced prostatic hyperplasia in Sprague-Dawley rats. *Journal of Pharmacy and Pharmacology,* 995-999.

Arunima, S., & Rajamohan, T. (2013). Effect of virgin coconut oil enriched diet on the antioxidant status and paraoxonase 1 activity in ameliorating the oxidative stress in rats – a comparative study. *Food & Function,*1402-1409.

Bata, Sabrina. (2014) What Is Ghee? 8 Health Benefits Of Clarified Butter. *Medical Daily.*

Bernal, M.D., Ph.D., J. (n.d.). Thyroid Hormones in Brain Development and Function. *Professor of Research Instituto De Investigaciones Biomedicas, CSIC-UAM Center for Biomedical Research On Rare Diseases (CIBERER) Arturo Duperier 4, 28029 Madrid, Spain.*

Blythman, Joanna (6 Feb 2013). At last, the truth: Butter is GOOD for you - and margarine is chemical gunk. *Published by Associated Newspapers Ltd*

*Part of the Daily Mail.*

Bowen, R. (2009, August 1). Physiologic Effects of Insulin. *Colorado State University.*

Calorie intake in relation to body-weight changes in the obese. Kekwick, A, Pawan, GL. The Lancet, 1956 Jul 28;271(6935):155-61.

Cardiovascular diseases (CVDs). (March 2013). *World Health Organization.*

Catalfo, G., Alaniz, M., & Marra, C. (2008). Dietary lipids modify redox homeostasis and steroidogenic status in rat testis. *Nutrition,* 717-726.

Coconut Oil: A Scientific Perspective. (2014). *Cure Alzheimer's Fund.*

Correction: Association of Dietary, Circulating, and Supplement Fatty Acids With Coronary Risk. *Ann Intern Med.* 2014;160(9):658. doi:10.7326/L14-5009-9

Courteney, Hazel. (26 Aug 2008). They were healthier than us - and even lived longer. So should we all copy the Victorian diet? *Associated Newspapers Ltd Part of the Daily Mail.*

D'Agostino, R., & Kannel, W. (n.d.). Epidemiological Background And Design: The Framingham Study. *Proceedings of the American Statistical Association Sesquicentennial Invited Paper Sessions-1989 & 1988.*

Dean, MD, W., & English, J. (2013). Beneficial Effects on Energy, Atherosclerosis and Aging. *Nutritionre.*

*Debmandal, M., & Mandal, S. (2010). Coconut (Cocos nucifera L.: Arecaceae): In health promotion and disease prevention. Asian Pacific Journal of Tropical Medicine, 241-247.*

Dhiman, T., Anand, G., Satter, L., & Pariza, M. (1999). Conjugated Linoleic Acid Content of Milk from Cows Fed Different Diets. *Journal of Dairy Science,* 2146-2156.

Effects of dietary fat and fiber on plasma and urine androgens and estrogens in men: a controlled feeding study. Dorgan JF, Judd JT, et al. American Journal of Clinical Nutrition, 1996 Dec;64(6):850-5.

Esterhuyse, A., Truter, E., & Oguntibeju, O. (2009). Red palm oil: Nutritional, physiological and therapeutic roles in improving human wellbeing and quality of life. *Br J Biomed Sci., 66*(4), :216-22.

Evangelista, M., Abad-Casintahan, F., & Lopez-Villafuerte, L. (2014). The effect of topical virgin coconut oil on SCORAD index, transepidermal water loss, and skin capacitance in mild to moderate pediatric atopic dermatitis: A randomized, double-blind, clinical trial. *International Journal of Dermatology,* 100-108.

Ferdman, Roberto. (2014). The War Against Butter is Over: Butter Won. *Quartz Magazine.*

Fife, B. (n.d.). Conquering Alzheimer's with Coconut Ketones. *Coconut Research Center.*

Fife, B. (n.d.). RED PALM OIL: A Daily Dose of Vitamins from A Cooking Oil. *Coconut Research Center.*

Ganzel, Bill. New Deal Farm Laws. (2003). *New Deal Farm Programs Change American Agriculture.*

Gasior, M., Rogawski, M., & Hartman, A. (2006). Neuroprotective And Disease-modifying Effects Of The Ketogenic Diet. *Behavioural Pharmacology,* 431-439.

Health and Nutritional Benefits from Coconut Oil: An Important Functional Food for the 21st Century. Presented at the AVOC Lauric Oils Symposium, Ho Chi Min City, Vietnam, 25 April 1996.

Hibbeln, J., Nieminen, L., & Lands, W. (2004). Increasing homicide rates and linoleic acid consumption among five western countries, 1961–2000. *Lipids,* 1207-1213.

Hunter, J.D. Diet, body build, blood pressure and serum cholesterol levels in coconut eating Polynesians. Fed Proc 1962;21:36-43

Isaacs, C., Litov, R., & Thormar, H. (1994). Antimicrobial activity of lipids added to human milk, infant formula, and bovine milk. *The Journal of Nutritional Biochemistry,* 362-366.

J Invest Dermatol. 2009 Oct;129(10):2480-8. Epub 2009 Apr 23.

Ji, S. (2013). MCT Fats Found In Coconut Oil Boost Brain Function In Only One Dose. *Green Med Info.*

Johanna M. Geleijnse, Cees Vermeer, Diederick E. Grobbee, Leon J. Schurgers, Marjo H. J. Knapen, Irene M. van der Meer, Albert Hofman, and Jacqueline C. M. Witteman. Dietary Intake of Menaquinone Is Associated with a Reduced Risk of Coronary Heart Disease: The Rotterdam Study. (2004 Nov 1). *J. Nutr.* vol. 134 no. 11 3100-3105.

Kabara JJ. Fatty acids and derivatives as antimicrobial agents -- A review, in The Pharmacological Effect of Lipids (JJ Kabara, ed) American Oil Chemists' Society, Champaign IL, 1978.

Ketogenic diet fights depression and bipolar disorder and aids weight loss. (2014, March 25) *AXS Digital Group LLC d/b/a Examiner.com.*

Lemieux, H., Bulteau, A., Friguet, B., Tardif, J., & Blier, P. (2011). Dietary fatty acids and oxidative stress in the heart mitochondria. *Mitochondrion,*97-103.

Lindeberg, S and Vessby, B. Fatty acid composition of cholesterol esters and serum tocopherols in Melanesians apparently free from cardiovascular disease - the Kitava study. Nutr Metab Cardiovasc Dis, 1995; 5: 45-53.

Lindeberg, S, Nilsson-Ehle, P, and Vessby, B. Lipoprotein composition and serum cholesterol ester fatty acids in nonwesternized Melanesians. Lipids, 1996; 31: 153-8.

Lindeberg, S, Nilsson-Ehle, P, Terént, A, Vessby, B, and Scherstén, B. Cardiovascular risk factors in a Melanesian population apparently free from stroke and ischaemic heart disease — the Kitava study. J Intern Med, 1994; 236: 331-340.

Lorgeril, M., & Salen, P. (2012). New insights into the health effects of dietary saturated and omega-6 and omega-3 polyunsaturated fatty acids. BMC Medicine, 50-50.

Lundell, D. (2013, December 8). Heart surgeon declares on what really causes heart illness. *Tuned Body.*

Malakoff, P., & Zucolella, G. (n.d.). Ghee – An Ayurvedic Perspective. *Amrita Veda.*

*Malhotra, A. (2013). Saturated fat is not the major issue. BMJ, F6340-F6340.*

Marina, A., Man, Y., Nazimah, S., & Amin, I. (2009). Antioxidant capacity and phenolic acids of virgin coconut oil. *International Journal of Food Sciences and Nutrition,* 114-123.

Micha, R., Wallace, S., & Mozaffarian, D. (2010). Red And Processed Meat Consumption And Risk Of Incident Coronary Heart Disease, Stroke, And Diabetes Mellitus: A Systematic Review And Meta-Analysis. *Circulation,*2271-2283.

Mendis, S. Coronary heart disease and coronary risk profile in a primitive population. Trop Geogr Med 1991;43:199-202.

Mozaffarian, D., Aro, A., & Willett, W. (2009). Health Effects Of Trans-fatty Acids: Experimental And Observational Evidence. *European Journal of Clinical Nutrition,* S5-S21.

Nakatsuji, T., Kao, M., Fang, J., Zouboulis, C., Zhang, L., Gallo, R., & Huang, C. (n.d.). Antimicrobial Property of Lauric Acid Against Propionibacterium Acnes: Its Therapeutic Potential for Inflammatory Acne Vulgaris. *Journal of Investigative Dermatology,* 2480-2488.

Nevin, K., & Rajamohan, T. (2009). Wet and dry extraction of coconut oil: Impact on lipid metabolic and antioxidant status in cholesterol coadministered rats. *Canadian Journal of Physiology and Pharmacology,*610-616.

Ogbolu DO1, Oni AA, Daini OA, Oloko AP. (June 2007) In vitro antimicrobial properties of coconut oil on Candida species in Ibadan, Nigeria. J Med Food 10(2):384-7.

Oguntibeju, O., Esterhuyse, A., & Truter, E. (n.d.). Red palm oil: Nutritional, physiological and therapeutic roles in improving human wellbeing and quality of life. *Br J Biomed Sci. ;66(4):216-22.*

Opposite effects of dietary saturated and unsaturated fatty acids on ethanol-pharmacokinetics, triglycerides and carnitines. Cha YS, Sachan DS. The Journal of the American College of Nutrition, 1994 Aug;13(4):338-43.

Overweight and Obesity Statistics. (October 2012). *The National Institute of Diabetes and Digestive and Kidney Diseases.*

Page, LB, Damon, A, and Moellering, RJ. Antecedents of cardiovascular disease in six Solomon Islands societies. Circulation, 1974; 49: 1132-46.

Philpott, Tom. A reflection on the lasting legacy of 1970s USDA Secretary Earl Butz. (4 Feb 2008). *Grist Magazine.*

Philpott, Tom. How cash and corporate pressure pushed ethanol to the fore. (7 Dec 2006). *Grist Magazine.*

Principles of Healthy Diets. (2000). *The Weston A. Price Foundation.*

Red and processed meat consumption and risk of incident coronary heart disease, stroke, and diabetes mellitus: a systematic review and meta-analysis. Micha R, Wallace SK, et al. Circulation. 2010 Jun 1;121(21):2271-83.

Reger MA1, Henderson ST, Hale C, Cholerton B, Baker LD, Watson GS, Hyde K, Chapman D, Craft S. (2004, Mar 25). Effects of beta-hydroxybutyrate on cognition in memory-impaired adults. *Neurobiol Aging.*

Salmon, W.D. and Goodman, J.G. Alleviation of vitamin B deficiency in the rat by certain natural fats and synthetic esters. *Journal of Nutrition.* 1936;13:477-500.

Sanmukhani, J., Satodia, V., Trivedi, J., Patel, T., Tiwari, D., Panchal, B., Tripathi, C. (2013). Efficacy and Safety of Curcumin in Major Depressive Disorder: A Randomized Controlled Trial. *Phytotherapy Research,* 579-85.

Shea, M., & Holden, R. (2012). Vitamin K Status and Vascular Calcification: Evidence from Observational and Clinical Studies. *Advances In Nutrition: An International Review Journal,* 158-165.

Sheldon Cohen, Denise Janicki-Deverts, William J. Doyle, Gregory E. Miller, Ellen Frank, Bruce S. Rabin, and Ronald B. Turner. Chronic stress, glucocorticoid receptor resistance, inflammation, and disease risk. PNAS, April 2, 2012 DOI:10.1073/pnas.1118355109

Shilhavy, B. (n.d.). New Alzheimer's Drugs Continue to Fail Where Coconut Oil Shines. *Health Impact News.*

Singh, A., & Purohit, B. (2011). Tooth brushing, oil pulling and tissue regeneration: A review of holistic approaches to oral health. *Journal of Ayurveda and Integrative Medicine, 2*(2), 64-68.

Siri-Tarino, P., Sun, Q., Hu, F., & Krauss, R. (2010). Meta-analysis Of Prospective Cohort Studies Evaluating The Association Of Saturated Fat With Cardiovascular Disease. *American Journal of Clinical Nutrition,* 535-546.

Solan, M. (2003). CLA: Can this fatty acid help you get thin? *Experience Life Magazine.*

Srinivasan, M., Sudheer, A., & Menon, V. (2007). Ferulic Acid: Therapeutic Potential Through Its Antioxidant Property. *Journal of Clinical Biochemistry and Nutrition,* 92-100.

Sugar restriction: the evidence for a drug-free intervention to reduce cardiovascular disease risk. *Internal Medicine Journal*, 2012 Oct;42 Suppl 5:46-58.

Tantibhedhyangkul, P. and Hashim, S.A. Medium-chain triglyceride feeding in premature infants: effects on calcium and magnesium absorption. *Pediatrics* 1987;61:537-545. http://dx.doi.org/10.1136/bmj.f6340 (Published 22 October 2013) Cite this as: BMJ 2013;347:f6340

Taubes, Gary. What if It's All Been a Big Fat Lie? (July 7, 2012). *The New York Times.*

Teegala SM, Willett WC, Mozaffarian D. (2009) Consumption and health effects of trans fatty acids: a review. Journal of Aoac International.

Testosterone and cortisol in relationship to dietary nutrients and resistance exercise. Volek JS, Kraemer WJ, et al. Journal of Applied Physiology, 1997 Jan;82(1):49-54.

The Impact of Stress: 2012 - *American Psychological Association.*

The Secret Sauce in Grass-Fed Beef. (n.d.). *Mercola.*

Thornley, S., Tayler, R., & Sikaris, K. (2012). Sugar restriction: The evidence for a drug-free intervention to reduce cardiovascular disease risk. *Internal Medicine Journal,* 46-58.

Time to fatten up our diets. (2007). *Harvard Health Letter.*

Tropical Oils. (2014). NYU Langone.

University of Iowa. (2014, June 17). Stress hormone linked to short-term memory loss as we age, animal study suggests. *ScienceDaily.*

Verallo-Rowell, V., Dillague, K., & Syah-Tjundawan, B. (2008). Novel antibacterial and emollient effects of coconut and virgin olive oils in adult atopic dermatitis. *Dermatitis.19*(6), 308-15.

20273334R00058

Made in the USA
San Bernardino, CA
04 April 2015